AF207051

# Rowdy Girl

# Rowdy Girl

## Confessions of a Vegan Cattle Rancher

*Renée King-Sonnen*

BLOOMSBURY ACADEMIC
NEW YORK • LONDON • OXFORD • NEW DELHI • SYDNEY

BLOOMSBURY ACADEMIC
Bloomsbury Publishing Inc, 1359 Broadway, New York, NY 10018, USA
Bloomsbury Publishing Plc, 50 Bedford Square, London, WC1B 3DP, UK
Bloomsbury Publishing Ireland, 29 Earlsfort Terrace, Dublin 2, D02 AY28, Ireland

BLOOMSBURY, BLOOMSBURY ACADEMIC and the Diana logo are trademarks of Bloomsbury Publishing Plc

First published in the United States of America 2026



Cover design by Jen Huppert
Cover image by author



Library of Congress Cataloging-in-Publication Data Available

ISBN: HB: 979-8-216-27835-1
ePDF: 979-8-216-27837-5
eBook: 979-8-216-27836-8

Typeset by Integra Software Services Pvt. Ltd.
Printed and bound in the United States of America

For product safety-related questions, contact productsafety@bloomsbury.com.

To find out more about our authors and books, visit www.bloomsbury.com and sign up for our newsletters.

*To Rowdy Girl, who gave me eyes to see animals never meant to be owned, consumed, or forgotten. They were meant to walk with us—not beneath us or for us. And to all who choose to listen when truth speaks, even if it costs them everything.*

# Contents

# *Figures*

# Acknowledgments

This book exists because truth insisted on being told—even when it would have been easier, safer, or more profitable to look away. It was carried forward by people who understood that bearing witness is not a performance, but a responsibility. To those who stood with me when the story was still unfolding, uncertain, and costly, I offer my deepest gratitude.

First, to my husband and partner, **Tommy Sonnen**. Our lives were irrevocably altered by the courage it took to question everything we had been taught. You walked with me through loss, upheaval, and reinvention, choosing conscience over convention again and again. This story is as much yours as it is mine.

To the animals—especially the cows—who trusted me long before I knew how to fully honor that trust. You were never symbols. You were teachers, mirrors, and living proof that love can dismantle entire belief systems. **Rowdy Girl**, and all who followed, changed the trajectory of my life and made this work unavoidable.

I owe deep gratitude to **Jane Velez-Mitchell**, who served as my sounding board through every chapter in the earliest days of this manuscript. You listened, questioned, encouraged, and—most importantly—urged me to write this book myself rather than hand my voice to a ghostwriter. Your confidence shaped everything that followed.

To **Morgan Kirchner**, thank you for guiding these pages through their earliest edits, long before this book found its way to a publisher. Your care helped the manuscript find its footing and discipline.

I am profoundly thankful to **Mitali Deypurkaystha**, who believed in this manuscript when it was still seeking its place and offered meaningful guidance before I pursued traditional publishing. Your discernment helped me understand what this book was asking to become.

To **Kip Andersen**: thank you for being the first to say—clearly and without hesitation—that this story had to be told. You were the first voice to say, *Write the book*, and that moment mattered.

I am deeply grateful to **Kameron Waters** for making the introduction that changed the course of this project. Your connection led me to my agent, **Ami McConnell**, whose steady guidance, clarity, and belief helped bring this book into the world with intention.

I am grateful to **Richard Brown**, my editor at **Bloomsbury**, for his thoughtful stewardship of this work. Your respect for its moral, spiritual, and narrative weight helped preserve its integrity on the page.

To **Jason Goldman**, producer of *Rowdy Girl*, thank you for recognizing the larger arc of this story and helping carry it beyond the written word.

I also acknowledge **Moby**, executive producer of *Rowdy Girl*, whose belief in this work helped others recognize its significance and lent credibility at a moment when this story was still asking to be heard.

I want to acknowledge **Drew Alexis**, who stood beside this work before it had a name, a structure, or a future anyone could see. Your guidance and steadiness helped bring Rowdy Girl Sanctuary into being long before it existed on paper. This work would not stand as it does without you.

I also acknowledge **Brett Christoffel**, who recognized the significance of a Texas cattle ranch choosing a different path and reached out in support when that choice was still unfamiliar and untested. Your belief affirmed that this transformation mattered beyond our own walls.

To the team at **Rowdy Girl Sanctuary**, past and present: thank you for the quiet, unglamorous, relentless work of care. You showed up in heat, mud, emergencies, and long nights. You held lives with integrity and tenderness, making both the sanctuary and this story possible.

I want to name **Lisa Browne**, whose steady presence through seasons of upheaval and perseverance helped carry this work forward. Your loyalty and unwavering belief sustained me more than words can express.

I also honor **Buddha**, my cat, who crossed the rainbow bridge but was beside me through every word of this book. You bore witness without language and anchored me when the weight of this story threatened to pull me under.

Beyond titles or roles, there has been a core circle—past and present—who walked beside me in spirit as much as in action. You held faith when mine wavered, steadiness when the path was unclear, and silence when words were unnecessary. This book was not written alone. It was carried, prayed into being, and borne through by a strength greater than any one person.

I am thankful to the donors, supporters, and allies who believed in this sanctuary when it was little more than conviction and risk. Your faith sustained lives—human and nonhuman alike—and made room for a future that did not yet exist.

Finally, to the reader: if you are here because something in you has begun to stir—because the old stories no longer satisfy, or because love has asked more of you than you expected—know that you are not alone. This book is offered not as a conclusion, but as an opening.

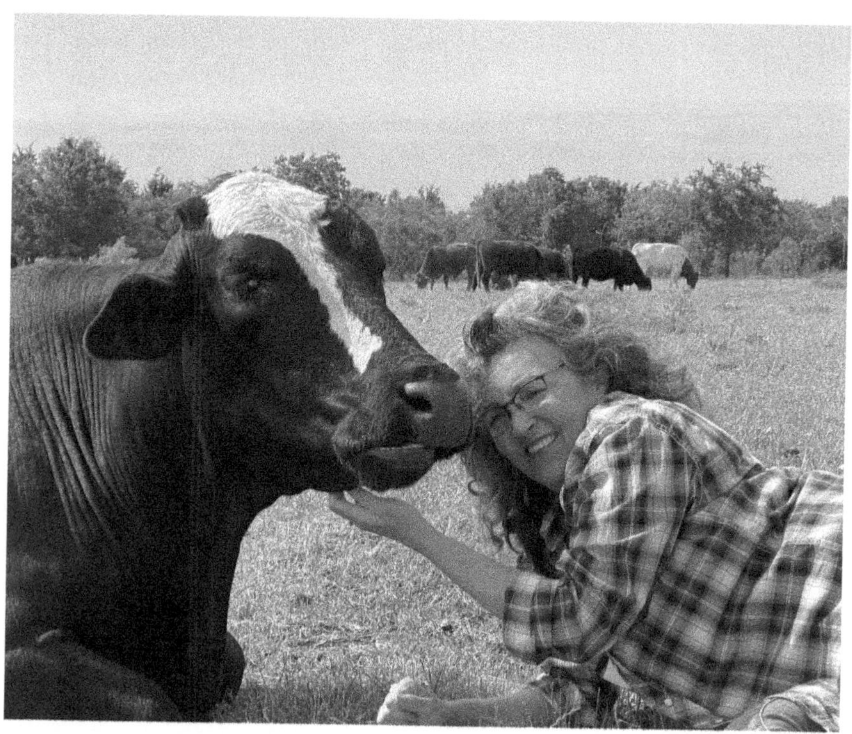

**Figure 1 Renée and Houdini.** *Houdini, Rowdy Girl's firstborn daughter. I nurtured her side-by-side with her momma, so she's always felt a little like my granddaughter.*

# *Introduction*

On October 31, 2014, I went vegan on a Texas cattle ranch. Everything I had been taught was uprooted, challenged, and threatened. All because of a calf named Rowdy Girl.

Rowdy Girl was my baby, my family, my friend, a rescued calf with the kind of eyelashes rodeo queens dream of. She taught me kindness, and in my constantly rebellious life, she steered me toward a great revolution. She and I have an intense and unique bond. I hear her, and she hears me. Not in the sense that we hear each other talking, but through intuition. Rowdy Girl awakened me. She continues to awaken me.

Our messages to each other come in waves, and they never stop. You see, Rowdy Girl and I are connected from the heart and soul, and whether I'm with her face to face, walking in a pasture, making breakfast, or asleep in my dreams, we commune. I can feel her through the air, no matter where I'm at. I can smell her, even at the perfume counter in the mall.

I've been told this is crazy; if it is, I wouldn't trade it for somebody else's idea of sanity. Once I accepted the fact that I was getting spiritual impressions from a cow, I went with it. It led me to a land of veganism, where animals are seen, not eaten. A place where animals are heard, not silenced, respected, not tortured. Where I love and where I am loved. This is a story about sanctuary for all creatures, me included. This is a story about betrayal, redemption, recovery, and revolution. This is a story about awakening and the evolution of a cattle ranch to the ultimate sanctuary for all creatures great and small—including me.

The Rowdy Girl mission has taken this Texas girl from Senate offices in Washington, D.C., to the bright, alive streets of Kathmandu. It has filled me at times with rage at our current food system and deep compassion for those in it. I am a product of the system, but I am no longer imprisoned by it. Most vegan-curious people I talk to don't think of themselves as imprisoned, but every time we consume animal products, we are taking in the violence, grief, and abuse they suffer; we are reinforcing a structure that keeps us from deeper peace, better health, true empathy, and freedom. My transition to veganism wasn't a dietary choice; it was a spiritual awakening, a rebirth, and recovery. It was the gift of desperation that broke me and brought me to my knees. I could not imagine the cows going to slaughter after I went vegan. I would have died for them. I would have stood between the red trailer and the cows to keep them from going to slaughter.

My fierce determination to save their lives *saved me.*

I came to the conclusion that there will be no peace on the earth without peace in our bellies.

At one time, I was terrified to speak these truths aloud. This way of life can be perceived as a threat to the cattle ranching culture and traditions. No cattle rancher thinks about going vegan. I had no neighbors, no friends, no people in my community to talk about what going vegan would mean, so I turned to social media. That's where I found Global Vegan Registry, and met Jeanne Westphal, who would become a dear friend and mentor as I grappled with the tension of being a vegan cattle rancher's wife.

She encouraged me to document my journey. And I listened. I made a Facebook page called The Vegan Journal of a Rancher's Wife. It was the biggest secret of my entire life. I didn't share it with anyone in my circle. (My husband didn't even know about it!)

I poured my heart into every post, as I wrestled with what to do next. Would I come home and find my cows had been sent to slaughter? That could not happen. How could I save them?

Thankfully, now I am able to share this story out loud, in these journal entries and in the following chapters. I'm living the life of a former cattle rancher turned rescuer out loud and in public! It's not a secret anymore.

I hope this book awakens the vegan in you and that you will reach out to me and let me be your next step into a life of freedom from the blood of animals.

I've included resources in the back of the book from vegan, spiritual, and philosophical giants. I encourage you to never stop learning and to use these resources to go as far down the rabbit hole as you need to get there.

# 1

# *Family and Friends*

*Ever since I was a little girl, I've been talking to animals. Sometimes I preferred the company of animals. I grew up with frightening violence in my home. But the animals I knew, they were never that way, never violent, never unpredictable, never seeking to dominate. Our pets brought me great comfort through their quiet presence and I could feel their thoughts and emotions, feel their sentience and their closeness to me. As a child, it was quite natural. As an adult, the ability to understand animals got quieter as life around me got louder and more busy."*

*May 12, 2025*

I grew up on a dead-end street in Jacinto City, Texas. It wasn't far from Houston, but it felt that way. Strays—kids and animals—roved the suburban streets. Dads went to work. Moms stayed home. Summer was hotter than a firecracker and long. I spent most of it outside with our cats and dogs.

The first thing that I knew about myself was that I loved animals. I always had a tender heart for them. Pets surrounded me at every stage of growing up. Even the most feral animals seemed to look at me with more curiosity than fear. My heart was wide open and receptive to the pain and suffering of those sweet beings in my care or stranded. I looked after them and they looked after me too.

My puppy dog, Checkers, was my best friend. She went everywhere with me and was as loyal as they came. We were inseparable. One beautiful day, when I was four, I decided to venture out alone with Checkers on my tricycle.

At the time, Momma was pregnant with my little sister, Jodie, and I didn't see anything wrong with taking off a few blocks up Flaxman Street to visit my Maw. Maw was Momma's mother, and I loved her something fierce. Don't ask me how I crossed the busy streets to get to the other side, but I did, and I felt safe because Checkers went with me.

I walked up the steps to Maw's house with Checkers at my side and knocked on the screen door. It was open.

Maw looked through the screen at me and then, with her mouth wide open, said, "Where's your momma?"

"At home," I said.

"Oh my God!" she screeched.

"Get in this house." Checkers and I went inside, and I started to cry.

"I just wanted to come and see you. I didn't mean to do anything wrong."

She called my momma, and I remember hearing them going back and forth in a frantic dialogue. Momma had been looking everywhere for me, and though she was relieved, she was not happy with me. Maw didn't drive, so Momma had to pick me up. I got a good talking to. She made me promise never to leave on my own again. She told me I could've been killed, run over, kidnapped, etcetera. She put the fear of God in me, but I never really felt like I'd gone somewhere alone. I had Checkers looking out for me. Momma didn't trust Checkers as fully as I did. And she had her reasons not to trust.

Momma had gotten pregnant with me at only sixteen, raped by my father in the cemetery where his first wife, Barbara, was buried. She married him because she was carrying me and because she was still a child herself.

My momma was pushed, shoved, or beaten every time my daddy came home from work or the beer joint. Once, he knocked her down in the bathtub while bathing, saying, "I'll kill you. Shut your f–king mouth!" She was five or six months pregnant with me at the time. His reasoning for knocking her down while standing in the tub was that she breathed too loudly.

Research shows that at twenty-seven weeks, a baby should start having regular sleep and wake cycles. A baby is fully developed at thirty-nine weeks. However, if startled at every developmental turn, you become wired to prepare for danger at every corner. It took me ten months to enter the world, and with that grand entrance came the next violent formative years of my life.[1]

My daddy remained a violent man, and violence, in a way, was his business. He ran King's Pawn Shop, and one of his biggest sellers was guns, lots and lots of guns.

Once he came home drunk and had my mother flat on her back in our living room with both hands pressing dangerously into her fragile neck. Her face was turning blue, and her gasps for air were diminishing.

"She's going to die," I gasped.

I ran into the kitchen and grabbed the biggest butcher knife I could find (I still remember the look, feel, and shape of the knife in my little hand). Anger, rage, fear, passion, *instinct* drove me headlong into the living room where I plunged toward my dad's back, with every intention of stopping him. I went one way, and the knife went the other. The fear and terror in her face and eyes were palpable. Something happened to me. I was prepared for battle. I was an animal, moved entirely by instinct. I felt the sanctity of mothers and children so deeply, so purely, that even then I would have died for her. She was so vulnerable, and every time I recognized that feeling in another being, I stayed close and made a point of looking out for them.

A stray tabby we called Momma Cat arrived when I was six or seven. She was a beautiful, wild-looking, tiger-striped feline who showed up at our house pregnant. I made it my business to ensure that Momma Cat was comfortable and had food and water. I couldn't wait for her babies to be born.

On the day the kittens arrived in our old beat-up and rickety garage, I was like a proud little momma myself. I was in awe of their small pink bodies, and I loved watching Momma Cat love and nurse them. She was so good at it. I had never seen love so natural. The old garage was termite-ridden and smelled of oil, laundry detergent, and musky dirt. The concrete slab was cracked near the washer and dryer. It was dirty. But with Momma Cat and her babies curled into each other, it was the most beautiful, peaceful place I'd ever been.

About five or six days after the kittens were born, I went into the garage, and my heart skipped a beat. Momma Cat was looking at me terrified, meowing frantically. A gallon can of paint was poured across the concrete floor, with big globs dripping all the way to the dryer. All four of her babies had been dipped in paint and dried to death. Their little eyes were not even open yet. It shattered my heart. I was frantic.

It turned out a neighbor boy, Mikey, did it. His momma didn't even reprimand him. Instead, she told my momma, "Oh well, kids will be kids."

*"Kids will be kids."*

I didn't understand. It wasn't a broken window, it was killing.

A mother had lost her children. It didn't matter to me what species of mother she was.

Every mother, including animal mothers, yearns for their children to be in their arms or by their sides. Every child needs their mother.

I wondered why my own momma didn't file charges on this family.

That boy came to our house and deliberately killed those babies. But violence was a part of our daily life. It was normalized in our culture and acceptable in our families. I can still see Mikey smiling behind his momma's apron.

Many years later, when my husband and I were cattle ranchers, we would lead the six-month-old calves into a red trailer and send them to a sale barn while their moms wailed loudly and grieved for days. They trusted us and we betrayed them. I never liked taking them to the sale barn, but like Mikey's mom, I shrugged it off. It was what we were supposed to do, or at least, what we knew to do. It was so ingrained. Our superiority to and dominance over animals is so deeply ingrained.

As a child, a little less conditioned, a little closer to my true nature, the hardness of my reality sent me repeatedly toward the softness of animals. They offered me friendship. They taught me lessons in loyalty and love that my own parents couldn't. I rejoiced in their births and grieved over their deaths.

When we found our beautiful Irish Setter mix, Ginger, lying dead on a grassy median miles outside of town, I covered her still-warm body with my own, laying my head into her gorgeous chocolate-colored shoulder with its strawberry blonde fur and streaks of copper running through the tips. I ran my finger down her long, pointed nose, and I wept as if I had lost a sister. I had. The loss was traumatic and affected me for a long time. I still feel her bouncy, loving, cuddly, and smiley presence.

The days that passed after the loss of Ginger were pure sadness. Tears would grip me when I saw her favorite ball, a stick she had been chewing on, and especially her bed. For a long time, I didn't want Momma to wash the dog bed, blankets, and towels that were all that remained of her scent. When I awakened every morning, I felt so much emptiness. Nobody understood. *But how could they not?*

I was "consoled" with the notion that animals don't have souls. For years, I tried hard to believe it. I'm so grateful that that lie didn't take hold. Ginger's soul will always be with me, along with other furry friends that have been part of my family through the years. They are a vivid part of my eternal memorial landscape. I'll never forget Ginger. I loved her, and she left an indelible mark of true love on my heart and soul forever.

Our instinct as children is to love and revere our animal friends. How many generations of children have fallen asleep with a teddy bear watching guard? How many cartoon heroes have tails? But our food systems defy that instinct. It teaches us to eat what we love. That humans are better than animals. And that some animals are better than others. What would it be like? Who would we be without this man-made hierarchy? If left to our devices, without this implicit permission, would a child ever murder a kitten? Would they mark the holidays with pieces of meat, or would it all look different?

Our whole family mourned over the loss of Ginger. I'm sure we had a plate with a piece of round steak or fried ribs for supper that night. We never once considered that the animal we ate could've had feelings and been loved by others like Ginger.

Why did I love my pets but eat farm animals? The only reason I can muster is that it was what I was taught. It's what I was programmed and conditioned to believe. I'd learned to like the taste and texture of an animal's flesh. I learned to eat their skinny neck and organs, like their liver, heart, gizzard, and other gross body parts, all mixed up in our Thanksgiving dressing every year. I still remember those soggy body parts wrapped in thick paper stuffed up inside the orifice of the turkey or chicken we were planning to roast.

I was accustomed to violence as a food group because, for generations, I was taught by my forefathers that it was normal. And it is normal, it's everywhere, but does that make it right?

# 2

# *Jesus, God, and All Things Holy*

*I began to feel the vibration, the frequency, and the beauty of being a bovine. I became one with them, and they became one with me.*

*August 28, 2022*

From as far back as I can remember, I've always had a deep connection to God, Jesus, and whatever power created this version of me in this lifetime. Even though I come from a Christian background and believe in Jesus, there's a part of me that senses I've been here before.

My earliest memories of going to church were at the Presbyterian Church in Jacinto City, Texas, where my Aunt Glenda was the organ and piano player. The church was a big, white building with a tall steeple and a cross on the very tip top. Vacation Bible School is one of my fondest memories of this period. I cherish those times and would look forward to the weeklong events where we delved into the life of Jesus, made arts and crafts, and ate cookies and Kool-Aid to our hearts' content.

I was about 8 years old when all that changed. Suddenly, we were thrust into the Church of Christ when my mother met a friend who convinced her this was the only way to heaven. I remember asking my momma, "Why are we changing churches?" She said, "Because we have to go to a church that Christ built, and the Bible says that Jesus said, 'Upon this rock, I will build my church, and the gates of hell shall not prevail against it.'" That is seriously the only reason.

From there, we were indoctrinated into the Church of Christ and taught that we wouldn't be saved and go to heaven unless we were members of the "church that Jesus built." *That* church was the Church of Christ. The scripture used to support this claim was Matthew 16:18. "And I tell you, you are Peter, and on this rock, I will build my church, and the gates of hell shall not prevail against it."

We were indoctrinated by attending many house meetings with the elders. Videos and biblical studies supported this to train us to be "true Christians" and followers of Jesus. We were indeed programmed to believe that the Church of Christ doctrine was the true and only way to get to Jesus and, thus, to get to heaven.

Having a musical instrument in the church was forbidden, so I grew up singing a cappella. The scripture used to drive this message home was Ephesians 5:19, which says, "Speaking to one another with psalms, hymns, and songs from the Spirit. Sing and make music from your heart to the Lord."

"How come we can't sing with a piano like we did in the Presbyterian Church?" I asked Momma one day. "Because a piano isn't allowed in the Church of Christ. No musical instruments were ever used in the Bible during worship service," she weakly explained. None of that made sense to my brain. There were cymbals, trumpets, harps, and so on mentioned in the Bible, but, by God, if it wasn't during an actual worship service, it wasn't allowed and was considered a sin.

The Church of Christ didn't believe that once saved, always saved, like the beliefs Baptists and most other nondenominational churches held. According to the Church of Christ, you could fall from grace and be damned to hell. So, I grew up believing that if I sinned and didn't get proper forgiveness, I could land in the lakes of fire.

Scriptures scared the heck out of me as a youth. I had to memorize verses like: "The backslider in heart will have his fill of his own ways, but a good man will be satisfied with his" (Proverbs 14:14); "But the Spirit explicitly says that in later times some will fall away from the faith, paying attention to deceitful spirits and doctrines of demons" (1 Timothy 4:1); "Take care, brethren, that there not be in any one of you an evil, unbelieving heart that falls away from the living God" (Hebrews 3:12). Whenever I recited these verses I would imagine myself as one of those characters in the Bible who committed these vile acts. Surely, I'd be thrown in the fire with them. As I'd hear these verses, I would feel the sensation of the flames burning up my flesh. I'd burn for the rest of eternity without relief.

I thought, *I'm never going to be saved. I'm never going to be able to measure up to what these verses are saying.*

So, when I started transgressing and committing sins, like kids do when they start experimenting with this, that, and the other, I felt like I was an unclean pagan. I was constantly begging God to forgive me and would visualize the blood of Jesus pouring over me so that I would be cleansed by the "blood of the lamb."

Thinking about this now, it makes me kind of sick to my stomach when I think of all those baby lambs that were sacrificed in the days of old, those that represented the coming of Christ. I'm really not sure where my brain lands on all that because I believe the will of man has *his* bloody hands all over the scriptures in the Bible that deal with animal sacrifice and the like. It's just plain demonic and reeks of satanic rituals.

I was always imagining the power of water. Jesus talked about water all the time. Sins washed away. I became fixated on the water. There must have been something supernatural about the waters—the Presbyterians didn't seem to get it. They only sprinkled their babies. However, in the Church of Christ, if you were not completely immersed in the water, head, nose, and every strand of hair on your head, you were not considered properly baptized in the Spirit and therefore risked damnation. No way in hell was a baby going to heaven if they were sprinkled and didn't eventually get properly dunked.

I would ruminate over verses like John 3:5: "Truly, truly, I say to you, unless one is born of water and the Spirit, he cannot enter the kingdom of God."

Romans 6:4 really kept me up at night. You have to be totally dunked in the water to be new in Christ. "Therefore we are buried with Him by baptism into death: that like Christ was raised up from the dead by the glory of the Father, even so we also should walk in the newness of life."

Well, there ya go! Gotta be born of the water regardless of which polluted lake it comes from.

Again, there are so many scriptures about baptism and how it represents being buried with Christ. The water represents the burial, and somehow that water represents the blood of Christ, and so on.

As a young girl, wanting desperately to please God and go to heaven and not hell, I constantly went up to the front of the church when Pastor Stanley asked us if we needed to repent for the remission of sins. I always felt like a dirty sinner, no matter how good I was. I remember going through a very dark time when I felt there was no way I would ever be let into heaven. I was just too much of a sinner because I'd been married so many times, had been a drunkard, a drug addict, and committed all kinds of what would be considered sexual misconduct according to scripture.

Especially so after my momma had a secret affair with one of the deacons of the Church of Christ, and everybody in Jacinto City found out about it.

That affair caused me and my family great anxiety at school because all my friends knew. I quit attending church and cursed the God I'd been taught to believe in for leading us into what I considered a true "lion's den of iniquity." Though the affair caused a really hard time in our lives, it eventually led my momma to divorce my daddy. When he learned about that affair, the beatings got deadlier, and my fierce resentment against God and the Church grew with each passing day.

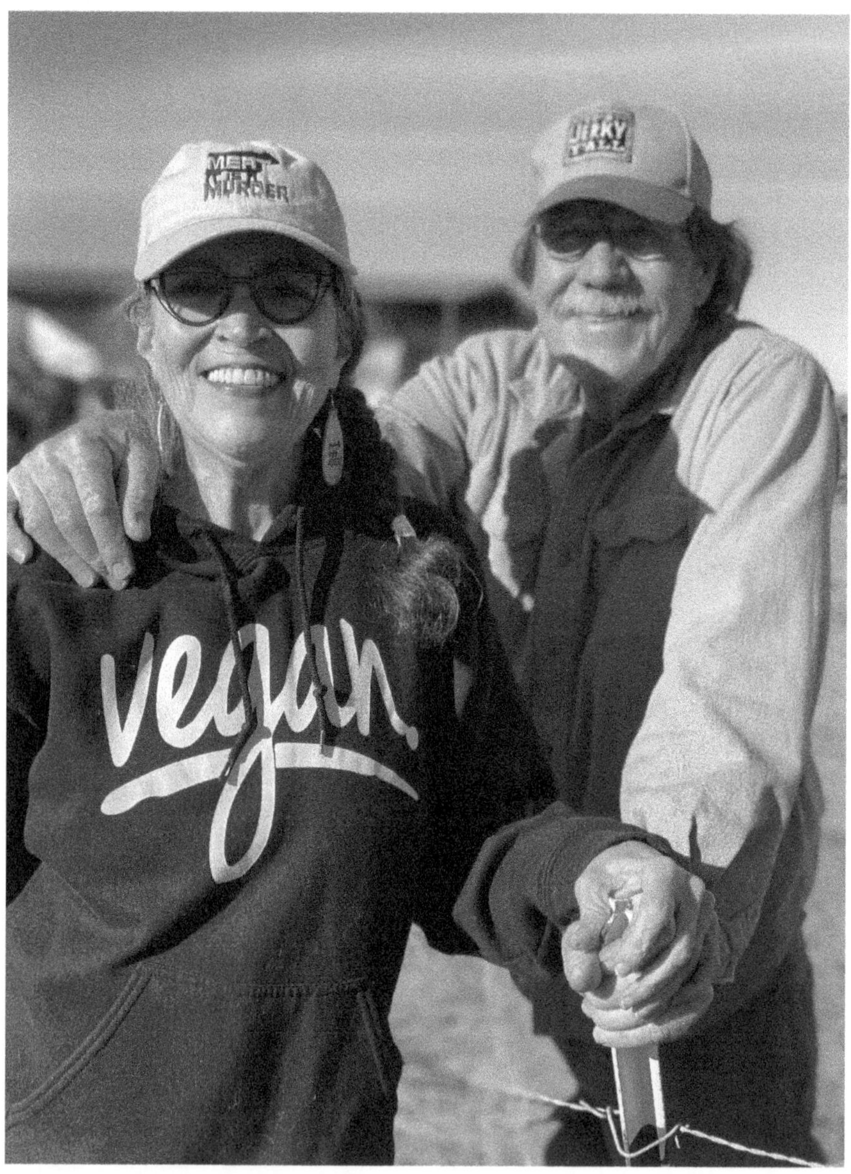


**Figure 2 Renée and Tommy.** *The couple who went from "raising cattle" to raising hell for the animals.*

# 3

# *Mine and Theirs*

*I used to participate in that which is not something I am proud of. That's why when I am asked to talk about it, I do. If my story can help anybody else decide to change the way they do things, then that's my service to humanity and to the animals.*

*October 30, 2022*

My father did not sexually abuse me. As depraved as he was toward my momma, he never touched me. However, without a healthy sexual blueprint, I didn't have a good impression of sex as an act of love. I had never seen my momma cherished and respected by a man. Love, as far as I knew, was violent. *Life* seemed violent, in large ways and small ones too—war, racism, sexism. The things we thought and said and ate—it was all violence. It all felt gruesome and destructive. Really, it wasn't surprising that I became destructive too.

The next chapter of my young life was filled with defiance at every turn. I defied all aspects of authority. I started drinking and drugging at an early age and was hell-bent on self-destruction. I put myself in more near-death situations than I could count. By age 15, I was an alcoholic and an addict. I went from one relationship to another, seeking someone to save me from inner torment. I was cruel to myself so that the rest of life's cruelties wouldn't come as such a shock.

My momma never loved my daddy. She told me the sex they had was always rape. I would beg her to leave him. Then, the violence escalated.

The final event was when I was 10 years old at my daddy's pawn shop. My siblings (Randy and Jodie) and Momma and I had just returned from a movie theater where we watched *Swiss Family Robinson*. It was a great movie, and I was still in the fantasy of it all when we got home to the final nightmarish chapter of my momma and daddy as a married couple.

My daddy was angrily speaking Spanish in the back office, and the next thing I knew, he came rushing into the living room and began questioning my mom with violent and obscene accusations. My brother and sister fled the scene as usual, and I stayed to defend against what I knew would become another violent attack on my mom.

I remember she wore houndstooth, black-and-white pedal pushers, black flats, and a starched white sleeveless blouse. Her hair was in her classic ringlet ponytail. I remember how beautiful and innocent my mom always looked before my dad bloodied her face and beat her fragile body.

Defenselessly, she would let him beat her, drag her, whip her. Over and over again, he would bloody her face until she was unrecognizable. I remember screaming at the top of my lungs for him to leave her alone. I remember telling him over and over that I hated him. Vaguely, I recall my brother and sister peeking around the hallway at this bloody scene that would become the finale of our life as a family.

My daddy had my momma's ponytail wrapped around his fist in one hand, and he beat her mercilessly with the other. Blood was everywhere. Her white blouse was soaked in it, as were her pants and shoes. In between blows, he glared at me with a crazed look I'll never forget and said, "Take one last look at your momma because you will never see her alive again." Over and over, he said this as he dragged her and a carbine rifle out of the house.

His car sped down the road, and they were gone for what seemed like hours. I huddled with Randy and Jodie, not knowing what would happen next. I heard the car come back, and my heart was beating out of my chest.

*I'm 10 years old, y'all. I'm wired to combat violence against the defenseless. That is how I'm f-cking wired!*

Daddy burst through the door dragging my momma by her hair, and dumped her in the middle of the living room. He went to the back office and once again was on the phone yelling and screaming in Spanish at someone.

My bloodied, defenseless momma came to me, gripped my shoulders, and looked into my eyes with the terror of someone running for their very life.

"Renée, your daddy is going to kill me," she said frantically. "He shot up the pawn shop. He aimed it at me several times and then shot up into the ceiling. I have to leave right now, or he will kill me. Take care of your brother and sister. I love you, and I promise I'll be back."

The fear and terror in her face and eyes were palpable. At that moment, something happened to me. I went numb and prepared for battle. I would endure whatever I had to in order to see my momma again. She left and there was silence. My daddy was furious. I later learned after we reunited with Mom that she jumped ten chain link fences and tore her houndstooth pedal pushers to shreds to escape. We didn't see her for two weeks.

My dad hid us out in sordid triple-X hotels. During those two weeks, my momma managed to get a restraining order and file for divorce. I'll never forget the moment when I saw my momma coming to get me in Mrs. Heuberger's fifth-grade class. My head was on my desk when I heard Mrs. Heuberger say, "Renée, someone is here to see you." I looked up and ran into the arms of my mother. That reunion will forever be etched into the wiring of my mind.

From there, I became very rebellious. I was blacking out drunk in my freshman year of high school. At 16 years old, I was raped at a high school party after too much alcohol and the downers that went with it. I was barely lucid at the time. I wish I didn't remember a thing, but I do. A popular football player did it. Other schoolmates stood around watching and cheering him on. The next day at school, he looked at me and smiled. It was an evil, vampiric smile, and I was so ashamed. It was humiliating. But at the time, shame seemed intrinsically tied to womanhood. After all, the same thing had happened to my own mother. I was a product of violation. I didn't hate him for doing what he did, not all the way anyhow, the same as I didn't hate my daddy.

After my mom and dad divorced, I went through a lot of emotional turmoil. I couldn't tell whether or not I wanted to spend time with him. Some days were better than others. We went through long periods where I didn't see or speak to him. These were followed by a yearning to know him. It was always a love/hate relationship.

We were both alcoholics, and he encouraged my escapades, calling me a "chip off the old block." Eighteen was the drinking age back then, so Daddy and I had a good ol' time in places like the Canary and the Shadow Club. We started talking about owning a nightclub of our own. Daddy bought one, and we called it the Coconut Grove.

I moved into one of the shabby little apartments behind the Coconut and became the bar manager and the band's singer. My alcoholism and drug addiction really took root at this time.

Daddy and I laughed and fought in equal measure, loudly. One night, he made me so angry, I stormed out of the Coconut around 2:00 a.m., walking down the feeder road of I-10 and Nimitz. I was wearing a beautiful cowboy hat with peacock feathers adorning the rim. I loved that hat. That was the last thing I remembered—how much I loved that hat.

When I came to, on the floor of a townhouse the next morning, my vagina was sore and I was bruised all over the inside of my legs, arms, and face.

It was cold and raining as light pierced through the tall windows without curtains.

*Where am I?* I wondered. As my eyes, ears, and sense of smell came into focus, I saw my jeans were inside out and across the room. There were beer cans, cigarettes, and clothing all around me. Naked men whom I didn't know were passed out and snoring.

Little dream-like bits of the night came back to me. I'd been raped.

My starched, long-sleeved, buttoned-down Western shirt had all the buttons ripped off. My bra was around my waist. Slowly, I looked around the room for my hat. It was nowhere to be seen. I could hear snoring upstairs, too. How many men had violated me?

My heart was pounding out of my chest as I squirmed to stand up and get the hell away as fast as possible. Without a peep, I dressed, tightly tying my buttonless western shirt at the waist, and left without a clue where I was, only knowing I had to run. I cried out loud as I tore down the street without my hat, the cold rain whipping and stinging my cheeks.

I ran until I found a place I knew. It was a neighborhood icehouse that Daddy and I had visited numerous times. They were just opening their doors. It was 11:00 a.m. I went straight up to the bar and started drinking again; instead of reporting the rape, I set out to drink the memories away. For a while I thought I had succeeded. I buried the trauma and kept on moving, just like Momma had and so many women before her—violence, violation, suffering, silence.

For years, the memories of those nights haunted me. I buried them the best I could.

One night, years later, I stumbled on a video segment about dairy production. I immediately felt sick to my stomach.

The program described the brutal process of forced insemination. It showed what looked like a metal rod that would be forced repeatedly into the animal. I learned that female cows, pigs, and turkeys were routinely violated to fuel the breeding conglomerates that treat them as "food." I got lightheaded watching it.

The memories came at me like a wave. The feminine is systemically debased and abused in our society. As women, we know this, we see it daily, but until that moment, I'd never thought about female animals. It's a convenient illusion to believe that a dairy cow doesn't feel the suffering and degradation. Good people, including myself, were eating and drinking the commodities of abuse packaged and sold as food. I was mortified. It was a revelation. It felt like neon lights going off in my brain.

I guess when you've experienced vulnerability, terror, and betrayal at that level, like I have, it becomes easier to identify, empathize, and recognize it in others—*even a dairy cow.*

I had always felt deeply for animals, but something deepened in me during this time, even as I spiraled out of control. I started to consider how farm animals felt in the blood-stained hands of farmers and ranchers. Farmers coax their herds into trusting them, but in the end, we betray them over and again. Don't we lead them to slaughter and lull them to sleep with green pastures and sweet feed? Don't we even name some of them and treat them well up to the moment of reckoning, only to violate their trust entirely by leaving them in a sale barn to be bought and sold for slaughter?

That's what *we* did.

We are a species capable of using and violating each other without thinking twice. Why was I surprised to find that animals suffer the same dishonor every second of the day by humans like me claiming to know so much about love, light, and faithfulness? The violence was happening all around me—*in spite of my so-called love, light, and faithfulness.*

What happens to these animals has consequences for us and how we treat each other. Why should anyone be shocked about what happened to me or others like me when we treat innocent animals just as bad or worse? We live in a world of normalized violence, sexual exploitation, and extreme betrayal, and it has deep roots in animal agriculture. If we stopped commodifying, exploiting, and using animals, maybe we could end the betrayal and violence we bestow on our human families and friends.

Not surprisingly, my alcohol and drug addictions spiraled out of control over the next few years. As I grew into a young woman, I used men and women for money and went through lovers like water. I wasn't proud. I had no sense of self as a lady. I was a chameleon who became what she needed to become—*in order to survive.* I was living in a system that promoted cruelty, so of course, cruel is what I became.

# 4

# The Lost Years

*Eating the chopped up bodies of beings is normalized violence.*

*August 28, 2022*

Around 1984, I was living it up at a southwest Houston nightclub when I met an Iranian man who owned a company called the European Car Connection. We hit it off. He was married, emotionally unavailable, and lots of fun. He hired me to work for him, and the next thing I knew, I found myself living the life of the rich and famous. Any European car I wanted to take home was at my disposal—Mercedes, Porsche, Jaguar, Rolls-Royce, you name it.

Anyway, during this time, I was lost and lacking a moral compass. That's when my grandmother—*Maw*, as I called her—rang me up. She told me about this family in Lake Livingston who had an old-time gospel country and western family music show. I still remember her voice on the other end of the phone. She was a Calvary Baptist all her life and prayed for me every day. Her prayers were answered, but not in the way she thought they would be.

"Renée," Maw hummed.

> I've been praying for you, Hun, and I know you are supposed to meet this godly family up here in Lake Livingston. They are a family of six, Jeanette, Dave, Mike, Ronald, Valerie, and Pamela Tucker. They all sing and play the best gospel and country music, Renée, and I know you would love them. I'd love to introduce you to them and see you sing with them.

Something was calling me to go. I loved my Maw so much. She was one of my biggest rocks growing up, and she always believed in me no matter how far down I slid. She loved Jesus like nobody's business and prayed without ceasing, she did. I decided to travel to Livingston to meet the Tuckers and to see my Maw.

As soon as I was introduced to this family, I felt a kinship with them. They welcomed me and treated me like part of the family. I was instantly brought into the fold, singing all the great gospel and country classics with them. After a few days of being in their company, I was once again *born again*, as we say, saved and redeemed from all my vile ways and promiscuousness. I was a new creature in the Lord. What started out as an overnight stay turned into a two-week visit. I later learned I had been indoctrinated into a cult and didn't even know it.

The Tuckers looked like Pentecostals but were known as Primitive Baptists. They wore long dresses, didn't cut their hair, wore no makeup, and were very modest. They spoke when spoken to, and the men represented Christ in the house. I felt reborn in their presence, and the way my life was going, I needed to be reborn. I quickly made plans to move in and be part of their ministry. Needless to say, I lost my job at the European Car Connection, but I didn't care. I was on my way to becoming part of the Tucker family.

The Tucker family lived in a small town in central Texas called Round Rock. Dave, the head of the house, followed me to my apartment in southwest Houston to help me pack up my belongings.

When we started boxing everything up, Dave was in another world. It was odd as all hell, but I didn't question it too much. After all, I knew men to be more crazy than not. He was loudly ranting one Bible verse after the other as I continued to pack my clothes and essentials. Suddenly, Dave put his hands on my shoulders and looked me in the eyes.

"Do you trust me?" he said.

"Yes, I trust you with my life," I said, because I did. He was a man of God, and this was my chance to begin again. Dave and his "godly" family touched me deeply. I was always searching for a family that was godly and loving. I yearned for a connection to a family that exuded biblical principles so I could have some structure and a template for how to be a loving family member. I didn't know how it was supposed to be—but I thought *this has got to be it.* I mean my Maw even recommended this family to me! I thought her prayers were answered. But this man, a preacher man, used this moment to strip my psyche of any innocent perception of who I thought he and his family were.

He asked me to sit on the carpet with him. My bed and other belongings were all packed in his truck. As we sat there, he began to fondle my hair and look into my eyes, quoting Bible verses that led me to believe that I was to be his spiritual bride. I could no longer have sex with anyone else but him, he said. He was to represent Christ, and I was to be his bride. In this way, all of my former transgressions would be forgiven, and I would be considered white as snow. I felt like I was being compelled to lay down and let this man christen me as his spiritual bride. As he penetrated me, I cried. But he said he did it in the name of God and Jesus!

It felt wrong. Like a trespass. Just as it had every time before. Yet, somehow, I shut it all out and believed him.

Dave let me gain trust in him and his family, came to my apartment and helped me clear it out, putting everything I owned in his truck. Then he took the last thing I had away from me—my innocent trust and my newfound faith.

What else was I to do?

The smell of Camel cigarettes and black coffee was the last thing I remembered as I succumbed to his will, allowing him to possess me, body and soul. A small part of me knew there had to be another way to live, to believe.

I lived with the Tucker family over the next few months, working in their garden and learning how to be a "proper lady" in the kitchen and in their family. My days were consumed with reading the Bible, prayer, and writing. I wasn't the only one in the house he was abusing.

On one occasion, I walked in on Dave to find his hands under the covers of his two young daughters, Valerie, 17, and Pamela, 14. They were in the same bed, side by side, and he was sexually fondling them.

After catching him, he cornered me in the laundry room with the dryer roaring as the rest of the family sang gospel music in the living room. He pressed his body angrily against mine, grabbed my chin with his cigarette-stained fingers, and through tight lips and yellow, crooked teeth, muttered into my ear,

"If you tell anyone what you saw, I will put you through a meat grinder, and no one will ever know what happened to you. Do you hear me?"

*Meat grinder*, the word was so vile. It rang out like a bell in my brain.

He pierced my eyes with a look that came straight from the devil himself. Terrified, I swore I would never tell a soul. Recalling it now brings back all that fear.

Fortunately, using my inner reserves of resourcefulness, I managed to survive and escape this dangerous situation through a loveless marriage to the bass player from the family band. That's a tale for another day. The most important thing is that I was able to escape.

Unfortunately, I turned my back entirely on God and the Church. I never ever turned my back on Jesus because I always loved Him with all my heart, but the ways of formalized Christianity were just too much to stomach.

Ultimately, I left it altogether and started studying other religions with a thirst for the "truth." There was no way that the God beating in my heart would ever turn me away. Something was wrong, and I was on a mission to seek God in all things. I knew the truth had to be somewhere other than where I was looking.

I studied all of it—including astrology, tarot, and other forms of the occult because all my life, I'd hungered for the understanding and affirmation that I could make my *own* decisions. I wanted a faith that made me stronger, more complete. I didn't want another lying, cheating, hypocrite of a man to tell me how to get to heaven.

"Studying to show myself approved," as the Holy Bible says in 2 Timothy 2:15, became the steering wheel of my spiritual quest. It was a journey that the Jesus I knew and loved was joyfully on board with. Would Jesus accept me, a wretched sinner, as His own? Would He ever accept somebody like me into the pearly gates of heaven? Would I be the kind of person who could leave this world better than I found it?

My spiritual quest led me to study all matters of the occult and the lost years and secret teachings of Jesus. In my Biblical studies, I came to understand that about seventeen years were missing in Jesus's life in the Bible. Why in the world would Jesus, the Messiah, not be correctly represented in the Bible during the years of His life when He was gaining knowledge and understanding Himself?

I became fascinated with these lost years. I still am.

Well, there were a ton of books out there on the subject, and for every book I read, there was always an evangelical critic who would say the writings were of the devil because they weren't *in* the Bible. Good grief, the Bible was first translated into English from the original Greek and Hebrew text by a largely forgotten scribe, William Tyndale (1494–1536). Fifty years later, the Bible was translated again under the auspices of King James. Traditionally, the original Bible was considered to have been dictated to Moses by God. The oldest extant (still surviving) interpretation of the Bible survives in a Greek translation called the Septuagint, dating back to the fourth century AD.

The criticism of blasphemy only fueled my curiosity. I will never believe that those lost years weren't important. Those searching years of my life as a young adult were vital to who I am today. After all my studies, I believe that the patriarchal translators of the Holy Bible didn't want us to know what Jesus was up to. If we did, we would also seek, as Jesus did during His lifetime, and there's no telling where we would end up.

As far as I could ascertain, Jesus was a truth seeker, an explorer who sought adventure, like me. It's absurd for the powers that be to act like those seventeen years of Jesus's life weren't important and just strip it out of a sacred text we are supposed to believe and follow to obtain eternal life. I wouldn't put it past the Jesus I love to have traveled and taught, and kicked a few tables over along the way when vulnerable people and animals were being tortured, confined, and hurt.

The sense of possibility in those lost years electrified me. I felt that I could forge my own path, that there were teachers and lessons far beyond school buildings and churches. I read voraciously. Thank goodness for library cards because I didn't have the money to be reading like I was.

After supposed preachers in the Christian faith severely abused me. I needed a break from the rules of man, so I sought a relationship with nature. I delved wholeheartedly into the world of Wicca.

When I stumbled upon the book, *Wicca: A Guide for the Solitary Practitioner*, I leaned all the way in. I was looking for a way to be alone with God, nature, and the laws of the Earth. This book helped me connect as an Earthling on this planet. It helped me to understand the elemental laws of earth, air, wind, fire, and ether. I don't practice it today, but it was a fork in the road of my journey. I believe Jesus was carrying me when I was healing from being so hurt by preachers, these so-called men of God who had warped my tender innocence with abuse, rigid rules, dogma, and masculine patriarchy.

He was carrying me toward light, hope, and true righteousness. I could feel it. It was the first time in my life, I felt truly seen and free. My beliefs grew, evolved, and flourished. And they were *mine*. They were not handed to me by someone else. There was no punishment for not believing. My mind was open. And truly, an open mind is the first step in cultivating authentic belief. For the first time, my own spiritual beliefs were taking root in Jesus's pure life-giving and fertile soil, not tainted by the violence of man.

I knew the results of that soil would yield the kind of fruit that Jesus talks about in the Book of Matthew: "By their fruits you shall know them."

I've been through more than a few books since those days and have remained a student of deep introspection. In all the spiritual works I've studied, the main constant thread is love, light, and compassion. Some of the very first books I studied about Jesus, God, and the Bible were: *The Lost Teachings of Jesus (Vol 1)*, *The Lost Years of Jesus*, and the *I Ching*. The stories in this literature gave me the tools I'd need to live my best life.

In the *I Ching*, for example, one of the principles is that all of life is in a state of change, in transformation, and nothing is static. Everything's flowing in cycles. They call it yin and yang. There's a biblical parallel here in Ecclesiastes 3, where Solomon writes: "To every thing there is a season, and a time to every purpose under heaven." Like the *I Ching*, the Bible teaches the inevitability of change and divine timing in our lives. These texts became respite for me. Eastern concepts like divine order and chaos helped me cope during this time. Then I'd open my Bible and read scripture about God's role as the author of peace and not confusion. These words comforted me as I traversed through immense chaos.

In the course of my studies, I learned about the Essenes, the ancient Jewish ascetic sect from the second century BC to the second century AD in Palestine. I wasn't shocked at all to learn they were vegetarians. They lived in highly organized groups and held property in common. The Essenes are widely regarded as the authors of the Dead Sea Scrolls. Jesus spent a lot of time in the wilderness, just like the Essenes did. His views were not in line with Pharisees or Sadducees of the day—but more in line with the mystical aesthetic worldview of the Essenes. He preached about love, the kingdom of heaven, nonviolence, and communal sharing—like the principles found in Essene literature.

Ultimately, I came to the conclusion that Jesus must have been vegan like we understand today. He loved animals and was an activist for all of God's creation.

If I had to say what I was at this stage of my life, I would call myself a "Vegan Christian" that leans into believing that Jesus was an Essene.

I began to struggle with traditional Christianity because of my "Vegan Christian" beliefs. How could the slaughter of animals be a part of anything "holy"? I saw how evil entered into the Bible, which caused good people to think that eating animals is righteous. *Even me!*

I really began to contemplate the verse Jeremiah 8:8: "How can we say, 'We are wise, and the law of the Lord is with us?' But behold, the lying pen of the scribes has made it into a lie."

Jeremiah was actively calling out the religious hypocrisy of the day. I was paying attention.

I took a hard look at my own upbringing. I never saw anything wrong with eating animals. Then it began to click. I had been indoctrinated into believing that eating the flesh of sentient beings was normal.

I came to the conclusion that evil is a corroding thread. I asked myself, how could anything good come out of a business that breeds, commodifies, and desecrates living beings to eat in the name of God?

Did God create us to be bred, born, tortured, and chopped to pieces for someone's so-called "food?" If not, why do we believe God created "farm animals" to be bred, born, tortured, and chopped to pieces for our food? Surely, this cannot be God's will. Is there anywhere in the Bible that orders humans to breed animals for food? I could find no scripture that literally says: breed animals so we can eat them. It's a human tradition, not a divine command.

In hindsight, I now know that humans have hijacked God's word and created their own messaging for profit, power, and pleasure. If we do not have to hurt another being to survive, why do we? There's one answer—conditioning, programming, culture, and tradition.

Seeking is deprogramming. In my sixty-eight years, I've done a lot of it. I've lived the lifestyle of a yogini (female yoga practitioner) and studied with yoga masters. I've been in the presence of the late Swami Satchidananda, whom I revere as one of my most eloquent, brilliant, and simplest guides.

I certainly don't subscribe to the notion that all teachers are wrong, but some can lead us astray, I'm sure of it. However, when we seek to know the truth, the truth finds us. From where I sit, seeking is always God's will for me.

My hope for my Christian brethren is that they take a moment to go deep within their hearts and "soul ponder" this for a while.

# 5

# *Birth of a Honky-Tonk Queen*

*When I met Tommy I was a singer who had my own band, I had a duo, and I performed solo. I also used to be one of the "star" vocalists with the Southwest Jazz Ballet, a touring dance company that had a forty-piece symphony band. We used to perform at military bases all over the United States. Tommy always said that for some reason I never made it in that world. Well now we know why—I'm supposed to be singing to the cows.*

*July 11, 2019*

The first time I ever sang in public, with a real microphone, stage lights, band, and a real audience, was when I was 17 years old and a senior at Galena Park High School. My best friend at the time was a girl named Terry, who convinced me to join her and the other "popular" girls in the Galena Park Beauty Pageant. This annual pageant was a highlight of every year, and 1976 was no exception.

There were thirty girls entering the pageant. It consisted of several competition categories—bathing suit, evening gown, interview, and talent. Our government teacher, Mr. Trammel, was the director. He was very fussy about the pageant having all the earmarks of those in the big leagues. Each entrant had a corresponding number, mine was ten, and during rehearsals, we had to line up and be appropriately choreographed during the show to qualify.

The competition's talent portion could be dancing, acting, or singing. My best friend, Terry, convinced me to sing because she always heard me singing in the car going to school and back. I agreed and chose our 1976 theme song, *Do You Know Where You're Going To,* by Diana Ross.

The only caveat I had was that I would not practice in front of my friends or Mr. Trammel. I would walk the stage with the microphone and mouth the words while the band played. I agreed to stand in my number ten spot so I wouldn't screw up the lineup, but I would only practice my song at home because I was terrified to sing in public. I thought: *What if I open up my mouth and nothin' comes out!*

On the night of the pageant, three hundred people packed themselves in to the auditorium, and the Galena Park band was in the pit warming up. I was nervous. The auditorium was buzzing with excitement and applause. I was waiting in the wings when the curtain opened. It was my turn to sing. I walked out in a long, flowing, red-sequined dress that my mother had made. The overhead lights and spotlight hit my face, and the band started to play.

I could see Mr. Trammel looking at me in the front row with a concerned look on his face as if he were wondering whether I might go mute. The moment I opened my mouth to sing, time stood still. Diana Ross asks the question, "Do you know where you're going to?" At that time in my life, I had no idea *where I was going to.* And I certainly had no clue that my voice would one day echo big for the animals. Diana's words tell a story of hope and no open doors. I had no idea what doors were going to open in the future and what rabbit holes were yet to explore.

I graced the stage as if I owned it and looked through the audience as if looking into another world. Mr. Trammel's eyes and mouth were wide open. The look he gave me was priceless. The lights were so bright I couldn't see everyone else. It felt like I was in my own little world, and the song became my own. I sang it as if I meant every word. I knew instinctively how to work the mic, walk the runway with lights out into the orchestra. I used the whole stage like a professional. I was so in the moment. It was like the first time I had ever met myself.

I was myself for the very first time. *And to think it was out loud and in public!*

When I finished, I got a standing ovation. I froze, bowed curtly, and ran off the stage to the dressing room, where I dove underneath a table in the corner.

My friends ran after me, in total astonishment. Here's a girl who didn't sing at all, and no one expected what was going to come out of my mouth.

Friends flooded in to the dressing room, telling me how good I was. The accolades were overpowering, and I started to cry.

I reached the top ten finalists and placed second in the talent division. Gosh, I couldn't believe it. That moment solidified my love for people, for making them feel good and happy. I learned I could be a conduit for joy, and the realization was powerful. My voice could change the mood of the room. When I sang, people listened. I could never, in my wildest imagination, believe that my little ole voice would cause that kind of reaction. But it turns out I just needed an opportunity to let it rip!

This moment solidified the transformation of a butterfly coming out of a cocoon.

I never had a problem owning the stage. It seemed I was born to be a performer. I had a voice and persona that people could hear and enjoyed listening to enough that they came back with friends. I would literally jump off that stage and into the audience's world on a dime to sing right to their woes, joys, and triumphs. A voice for the voiceless was born, and I had no idea it was happening.

When I left high school, I went on to sing at the infamous Gilley's and other various nightclubs and open-mic nights. I was the featured honky-tonk singer in my daddy's nightclub in Channelview, Coconut Grove, in the early eighties. I even won the talent round at Gilley's around 1981, singing the Hank Williams classic, "Kaw-Liga." It became *my* song. Everywhere I went, I was recognized and given the microphone to wow the crowd. I might've had confidence, but what I had even more of was passion. I loved singing; it mattered to me so much that all doubt was cast aside.

With every song and every stage, I grew surer of myself. Eventually, I decided that I wanted my own band! I wanted to go on the road! I didn't have any equipment, not even a microphone, but I could sing. *And I was convincing as all hell.* I called up a guy named Russ at the Houston Musicians Referral Service to see if he could help me get a band together to start gigging. After all, I was now a pro, I thought. Ha!

"Do you have any gigs?" Russ asked.

"No, I don't have a band," I said.

He laughed, "Well, you have a problem! Do you have any gear?"

"No," I said, and my heart dropped.

He chuckled, "Well, good luck. It sounds like you're gonna need it. The best I could do for you is to get some high school kids together to play with you in a garage band."

For a moment, I felt humiliated and defeated, but only for a moment. So, I thought, in order to get a band, I need gigs and equipment. Well, I reasoned, I could get the gigs. I'd been singing all over Pasadena and the Houston honky-tonk strips since the high school beauty pageant. They all knew me. I decided to tell a little white lie so that I could get the band together and get on the road. A girl's gotta do what a girl's gotta do.

I went to four nightclubs and booked six weeks' worth of work with bar owners. I convinced them all that I had a band, we were rehearsing, and we would be ready for the stage in a couple of months. My calendar was full. Four nights a week for six weeks at two hundred dollars per night. That was fifty-bucks per musician. Not a bad rate in those days.

All I needed to pay was a guitar player or two.

I called Russ at the Houston Musician's Referral Service again and told him what had happened. He was shocked.

"What?" he said. "You mean you booked Chipkickers without a band?"

Chipkickers was a well-known dance hall in North Houston that had live music seven nights a week. The owner, Bobby Joe, loved me.

"Yes," I said proudly. My heart was beating out of my chest.

"Well," said Russ, "You got bigger balls than most guys I know if you pulled that off."

We laughed and Russ gave me a list of musicians to call. He also started referring musicians to me since I had the gigs.

"Now, what about equipment?" he said.

"Well, I got the work, didn't I?" I said confidently. "Something will come up."

Russ was floored. "Girl, you are crazy. What if you don't get that equipment and you've made promises you can't keep?"

"That's not an option," I said, and I meant it.

The following days were filled with phones ringing and musicians coming over to rehearse so I could choose my band. I picked out the guitar, bass, and steel guitar musicians. I still didn't have any equipment, but nobody else knew that. A drummer named Richard Rivera rolled in from Nashville with a trailer full of equipment. He had been on tour with a country singer named Tammy Lynn and was back in town after the shows ended.

Richard came in to rehearse, and before he set up to showcase his drumming skills, I said, "What's in that trailer out there?"

He told me it was full of music equipment, lights, a soundboard, and all the cords and such to go with it.

"Wow," I exclaimed. "You're hired."

"You haven't even heard me play yet!" he said, puzzled.

"That's OK," I said, "Let's play, but you're hired anyway because I don't have any equipment, I have all these gigs booked, and we have to be ready to play in six weeks."

He grabbed a beer, shook my hand, and from that moment on, we were partners. In my mind, he was sent from God Almighty, an answered prayer.

As we sat drinking our Lone Stars, I thought about how crazy it was that I'd gone from a girl waiting for a man to tell her what to do, to a woman giving the orders. Singing had made me strong, brave, and rowdy. It taught me that when you have a passion, when you use your voice, you can change things in the world.

When I hired Richard for the job. Everything lined up. Not only did we have gigs, but we also had showcases. The band *Renée King & Wildcard* was born. Richard became not only my drummer but my stage manager, promoter, boyfriend, and booking agent. A honky-tonk queen *and* an activist was born.

My experience performing, singing, promoting, and public speaking has been the bedrock of Rowdy Girl Sanctuary's success. You don't convert a cattle ranch to an animal sanctuary in twenty-four hours by keeping your mouth shut. I didn't have a clue how I would do it, but I was determined as hell to make it happen. The ability to persevere through all hardships no matter what, to have the attitude of "the show must go on" whether there's a flood, a freeze, or a drought, the ability to stand firm in the face of adversity of all kinds and never give up, has been the defining mixture of ingredients that has grounded my footing in the animal protection community. It put me in the unique and unexpected position of being a voice for farm animals worldwide.

It is my deepest prayer that all the life skills that I perfected as a country and western honky-tonk queen on the road might be used as a shining light for the animals that need my voice. What matters to the animals that are screaming in silence is that we all use every ounce of talent, skill, and creative ability that we can muster to end their suffering and to shut down animal agriculture.

We have to get creative and be bold. Use what you've got! The animals are depending on us. Whenever I needed to have the Red Sea parted, God showed up. This has been my experience time and again.

If a small-town girl in Jacinto City, Texas, who grew up with nothing can make a difference, you can too.

# 6

# *Ahimsa*

*The whole system is indeed broken. Be a part of the solution, not the problem—choosing vegan is the only compassionate choice.*

*May 28, 2017*

In 1988, I started practicing traditional yoga after a nasty car crash caused me excruciating back pain. My injuries were debilitating and landed me in the emergency room repeatedly, barely able to move. I tried to live with it, but I would be OK one minute and in agony the next.

Once, the pain was so bad that I couldn't even blink an eyelash without screaming. I went off to the ER for (yet another) shot of Demerol. At the time, I was performing nightly with my band, and I wasn't one for canceling gigs, but I had no choice. I was devastated. Richard, my drummer and boyfriend at the time, finally convinced me to try a traditional Chinese acupuncturist in San Antonio. I was skeptical, but I would have tried anything to feel better at that point.

The acupuncturist kept me for three days. After that, my pain was gone. He told me he had placed almost three hundred needles in my body over seventy-two hours and that if I didn't start doing yoga, I was gonna die young.

He told me all about the body's meridians, made me a cup of bitter hot tea, and walked me over to a dozen charts of the various meridian channels. In traditional Chinese medicine, meridians are lines connecting acupuncture points. These lines are the passageways in which energy, or *chi*, flows throughout the body.

The acupuncturist laid sheets of onion paper over each one to show me where my energy channels were blocked according to each corresponding meridian. As he educated me, my mind started going back in time.

Somewhere along the way, in another life perhaps, I knew this stuff. It all felt true and familiar, though I had never been taught about meridians. I thought about where I was in life, drinking, drugging, dating all the wrong men for all the wrong reasons—though Richard was just fine. I was trapped in a cycle of self-destruction, carrying equal amounts of pain from my childhood, and, now, fear for my future.

The acupuncturist recommended a book called *Richard Hittelman's Yoga: 28 Day Exercise Plan.* Twenty-eight days sounded reasonable. I went home and started practicing. By the end of Day One, I was hooked. When I finished the book, I went ahead and started right over again. I did that several times, but I knew I needed a teacher to progress.

I started taking yoga classes at the former Yoga Center of Houston, studying with Yogi John Coon, both in the classroom and privately. From there, I received multiple certifications as a teacher, studying with M. T. and Roberto Mazzarella with Yoga for Every Body, Sandra Summerfield-Kozak, director of International Yoga Studies, and various Kundalini yoga teachers. I was eventually certified in Kundalini yoga. Additionally, I studied Ayurveda and received certification as an Ayurveda Practitioner.

I'm still an avid yogi. I've practiced Integral Yoga created by the late Swami Satchidananda. I've spent many weeks at the ashram in Buckingham, Virginia, in ten-day stretches of silence. I also love the Sanskrit and Gurmukh chanting and have a fond appreciation for the *Yoga Sutras of Patanjali*, the *Upanishads*, and the *Bhagavad Gita*. I've even owned two yoga studios: Breathe, Move, Relax, and Stretch in Lake Jackson, Texas, and Yoga and Performance by Renée. I was also a managing partner in a wellness center that included a yoga studio: Total Wellness Spa, in Dickinson, Texas.

What struck me most about yoga back in my early learning days was the concept of alignment. The practitioner is advised to align with the eight limbs of yoga. The first two limbs comprise what are called the *Yamas* and the *Niyamas* of Yoga. *Yama* means "self-control," and Niyama means "moral observance or personal habits." Back in my wild days with the Wild Card,

I was not aligned. I was hurting myself. The distance between who I was and what I believed was vast. I was addicted, dependent, and depressed. I knew I needed to find a way out, not just from my physical ailments, but my spiritual ones.

The concept of Ahimsa, nonviolence, not hurting ourselves or others, stood out. Apart from causing physical harm, I learned there were other forms of violence, such as mental and emotional violence. Feeding your body toxic food and feeding your mind toxic thoughts such as anger and jealousy are all types of violence. I had never thought about those things as violent, but they had certainly felt that way before.

In my mind, violence was Daddy bursting through the door, dragging my momma by her hair, and dumping her in the middle of the living room. It was her coming to me, gripping me by my shoulders, and looking into my eyes with the terror of someone running for their very life. I'd never considered my drinking an act of violence. I sure as hell never imagined my turkey sandwiches were hurting anyone. Heck, I thought they were healthy! But it all mattered, the way I spoke to myself, what I thought when I looked in the mirror, and the things I believed.

Interestingly, in all my years of yoga training as a student and teacher, I was never told that I must abstain from *all* animal products to satisfy Ahimsa. Vegetarianism was encouraged as a practice during teacher training modules, but at that point, I didn't feel that abstaining from animal products was something I should do for the sake of ethics. The other yoga practitioners I knew practiced, taught, and meditated, and then went straight to a barbecue over the weekend. In my Kundalini yoga classes, we were instructed to get a sheepskin to sit on as part of our practice. I paid reverence to my body by attending to the postures, the asanas, and breathing practices known as pranayama, but I nourished it with animals that were tortured and experienced agonizing deaths. Even when my physical pain was gone, my spirit remained heavy and I didn't know why. I continued numbing my emotions with alcohol for years, unaware that to fully live out Ahimsa, I would need to do more.

We truly are what we eat. When we eat violence, the subtle energies of that violence flood our system. My system was awash with terror, fear, and grief. There is another yogic term, *nadi*, which is pronounced "knotty." *Nadi* means "stream" in Sanskrit, representing a network of subtle channels through which our life force circulates. I was suffering energetically in every part of my being.

It's not like I did a downward dog and immediately got sober and stopped eating chicken, but something about Ahimsa changed me. It was the first time I paused and considered the harm of my choices, even the smallest ones, could cause. It helped me define violence in my life and helped me recognize the role I played in perpetuating it. It was the beginning of accountability, humility, and in many ways, recovery. Self-reflection is an important part of self-discipline. It's important for us all to take ownership over what we put into our minds and bodies, and what we project into the world.

It wasn't until I was 57 years old that I learned to be true to the first Yama of nonviolence. Ahimsa is my nature, and my nature loves and reveres all nature, including the meekest of all in God's animal kingdom. They are my friends, they are my family, and they are me. I've never been more content in my life than I am now.

Vegans frequently say, "The only thing I regret is that I didn't go vegan sooner." I've never been more content in my life than I am now.

To be free of culture, tradition, and familial loyalties that use and abuse animals is indeed the most contented feeling in the world. *That's true Santosha*, or "contentment" as yogis say. Santosha is the second Niyama of the eight limbs of yoga. (I could write a whole book on yoga and animal rights, but I'll stop there. For yoga-curious minds, there are more resources in the back of this book.)

I've been vegan since October 31, 2014. I have a rich prayer and meditation life. I'm free of death and suffering in my body. My physical form and *nadis* no longer represent a graveyard for the meaninglessly tortured souls of animals. I've become so sensitive to their suffering. I pray incessantly for their freedom.

I pray for your freedom, too. I awaken with prayer and meditation each day. Before I retire, I thank God for another day now sober, and for my vegan lifestyle that embraces all of God's creatures as worthy of life and reverence.

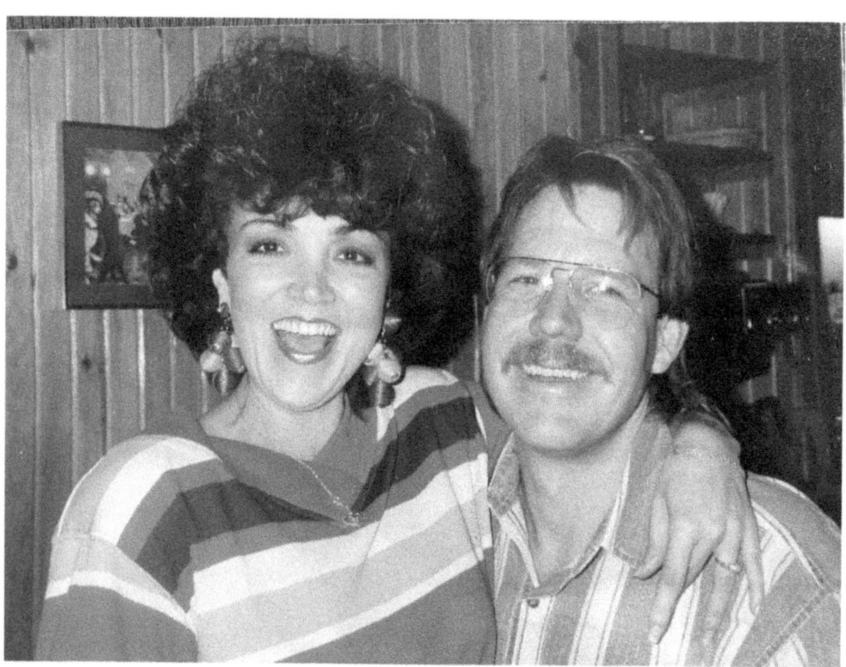

**Figure 3 The Past**. *Me and Tommy in the early days—back when my hair had its own personality, and he still believed life with me would be simple. Neither of us knew that love, loss, and a herd of cows would steer us into a destiny we never saw coming.*

# 7

# *Renée and Tommy*

*Now back to the "Unlikely Love Story" of me and Tommy. We've grown up together—we're still growing up. I wrote a song for him in the early 90s—it's called "When I'm Out of My Mind." God knows, I've been there a time or two with this man.*

*February 16, 2020*

I married Tommy Sonnen for the first time in April 1991. I was three months sober and performing at a Hilton nightclub in Lake Jackson, Texas. The night we met, I wore red spandex pants, a red satin-waisted blazer with white fringe dangling from the arms, and knee-high, white-leather cowgirl boots. I teased my hair out in an 80s "big" style, and I always completed my costume with a black-penciled mole just below and to the left of my ruby-painted lips, perfectly placed on my delicate chin.

Had I known then what I know now, would I have given him the time of day? I'm not sure, really. Or maybe there's another way to look at it. The wind in the air was right that night when he came strutting in the door at closing time. Unbeknownst to me, Tommy's best friend Robert told him that there was a girl at Michael's Club who wanted to meet him.

I did not tell Robert that I wanted to meet Tommy. Robert made that story up, trying to get Tommy to Michael's Club so that he could set us up.

With a spotlight on my face, I left the stage, walked to the bar, and sat right on his lap. He had on a pair of Wrangler jeans, spit-shined Roper boots, and a freshly starched Rocky Mountain long-sleeved shirt—with just enough Aramis cologne to make me wanna bury myself in his neck.

With all the seductive and sultry nuance I could muster, I took the microphone to his ear and started singing the Patsy Cline classic, *Crazy*.

The song choice was an omen.

That moment is seared in my consciousness. It brands the moment when our everlasting love took shape. We've had our ups, downs, and all-arounds, but we've always come back to North on our compass. Our chemistry is the magic ingredient in the Rowdy Girl movement. It's also caused a heck of a lot of drama.

Yes, indeed, the wind in the air was right that night, Mother Earth came out to play, and an epic love story was born. But I don't know if I'd call us a Fairy Tale. I was a full-blown, card-carrying alcoholic and had my own country western show band on the road. I didn't always make the best decisions. I was trying to be better, but I was getting worse. Tommy was a hard-working, hard-playing Texas man. He worked for Dow Chemical and had just got off the evening shift. The bar closed at midnight, and he came in right at closing time—just enough time to sweep me off my feet, and nine months later, we were married.

Before we got married, I started drinking again. Tommy didn't know how bad off I was. It all started with an innocent marijuana joint he'd saved up for a special occasion. It turned out *I* was that special occasion. Before long, I was tempting fate, mine and his. I was blacking out again. I got so drunk on our honeymoon in San Antonio on the Riverwalk that I barely remember it. Although I *do remember* eating at Dicks Last Resort, where the obnoxious staffers cussed us out while ordering our meal. It's part of their schtick. (Who knew this rowdy joint would be another omen for rowdy things to come).

We held it together until about 1995. I'd spent the better part of ten years performing on the road, and I was ready to take my career to the next level. I convinced Tommy to help me open *Renée King's School of Performing Stars* in Houston, near the Galleria.

In no time, I had over thirty students and had acquired a great gig in the Houston Astrodome during the Houston Livestock Show and Rodeo. The Rodeo was part of what it meant to be Texan. I attended it every year and met lots of people in the inner circles.

I hobnobbed my way into the right places, and before I knew it, I managed to have my students opening for headlining acts. This was huge, as huge as my big head. My drinking and my ego were both out of control. It wasn't long before I started adding some harder stuff into the mix. Pharmaceuticals, cocaine, and marijuana all paired well with my expensive martinis.

The Houston Livestock Show and Rodeo was a big success, and you better believe I celebrated that way. Tommy's company, Dow Chemical, was having a party, and I partied all those *businessmen* under the table. I made a complete ass out of myself by sitting in his big boss's lap, to the chagrin of his wife, I'm sure. She was there. If my vision wasn't doubled, I definitely would have caught a few dirty looks from her. I drank and drank, and allegedly threw quite a few dinner rolls across the room. The rest is, at best, a gleeful blur.

The following morning, I woke up fully clothed to a disgusted Tommy Sonnen. A wise man named Bill said we needed to have that moment of clarity.[1] I'd known things were out of control for some time. I'd never been the woman or wife I wanted to be. But that morning, my mind finally opened up to the fact that I needed help. I told Tommy to take me to the hospital to detox.

As we were traveling down Highway 332 to go to the Brazosport Hospital, an antique car show passed us. There was every type of old car you could think of in every color. I saw Model T's from the 1940s and Thunderbirds from the 1950s, those old-timey Sedans rolling past in what felt like slow motion. My world dissolved, and I imagined a simpler and easier time when those cars were the latest and greatest rides on the road. A time before I was even born. A time when I could be free from the pain of the present. Free from the alcohol, drugs, and insanity of needing to perform and to be "Miss Renée," to be OK.

I was admitted to the fourth-floor psych ward. It was supposed to be a fourteen-day detox, but when the doctors discharged me, I panicked. I could not envision a world where I could function as Miss Renée. I had thirty students, all depending on me to feature them in major showcases all over Houston. I was producing a thirteen-week showcase for the Houston Community College System, and had just finished a successful wrap up at the Houston Livestock Show and Rodeo—the biggest rodeo in the country at the time. My students had opened for major acts like Trisha Yearwood, Doug Stone, and Tracy Lawrence.

And through it all, I was there in the Houston Astrodome, in the dark, wielding my power, like the Wizard of Oz—conducting their performances through my own body. Oblivious to everyone else around me—thousands of them! I would move around the Astrodome like it was my own personal stage, sending my electric current through every student. I wanted to make sure my energy got to each and every one of them through every sound and nuance. I felt like they were an extension of me.

How was I supposed to command this kind of energy and encourage my students to go to the next level and "become the star you know you are," as my classes promised, when my own shooting star had burned out. How could I develop people's full potential if I couldn't even take a step outside?

I looked in the mirror—where was Miss Renée—the vibrant lifeforce with an enormous persona—who harnessed the forces of nature?

Countless times, I would stand on stage in front of my students and tell them to visualize themselves with the deep roots of a tree: "Go into the heavens. Ground yourself, root yourself. Now go to the heart of your being and pull that energy up from your feet into your heart. And when you open your mouth—just sing."

The irony is I had no roots at this point. I was so devastated. Where was that woman who could inspire students to go to their depths and reach for the heavens?

I was the classic Humpty Dumpty teeter-tottering on the wall.

I had no connections in my brain to inform my next step. I had no frame of reference for how to live without alcohol, drugs, performing, teaching, and producing. How do you do that as a fragile recovering alcoholic? I felt like a shell of a person. I had no roots in this new life. I was afraid to live.

Tommy was so excited that I was coming home. He had kept all my plates spinning for two weeks—telling my students and students' parents that I was sick.

I knew it was not possible to return home.

I spoke with the staff about checking into a halfway house, called The Right Step, where I could live for six months.

That initial conversation with Tommy didn't go well.

"You're not homeless. Why do you want to go to a halfway house? You have a home," he said in disbelief. He thought his marriage was over. How could he pay the bills?

Tommy picked up all the pieces of my entire world. He called every one of the parents to let them know that Renée King's School of Performing Stars was shutting down. It was such a blow.

Meanwhile at The Right Step, I lived among other recovering alcoholics and addicts and began to heal by unlearning everything I ever thought was true about myself. This period was brutal for Tommy, to put it mildly. He was crushed—lower than I ever remember him being.

My therapy was so intense that I regressed into a borderline personality disorder. Because my past trauma was so deep, the personality of "Renée" had to go to sleep, and "Holly" was born. I had to dissociate to survive—I could not identify with the abuse that Renée had endured for decades. The pain of Renée's memories was soul-crushing and mind-searing.

Even when Tommy would call to speak with me, I would tell the staff that Renée wasn't here.

"If he wants to talk to me, then he needs to ask for Holly," I'd say.

That took a huge toll on him.

Renée writes with her right hand, but Holly wrote with her left hand and had no problem doing everything her psychiatrist told her. While Renée was large and in charge, telling everyone what to do—Holly was quiet, submissive, and compliant. She became the ultimate poster child of recovery, and because of her past sexual trauma and violent upbringing, she had a challenging time reintegrating into society. After some intense art therapy with a psychiatrist named Dr. Busch, I slowly began to experience a rebirth. I was like a little child again. Eventually, the time came for Renée to come back. I was still vulnerable—like a child, insecure and scared to return to whatever "normal" used to be.

Our marriage couldn't survive my recovery. While doing my AA step work, I was inundated with the horrible things I had done while drinking. The guilt forced me to create havoc in my marriage. We sought counseling and couples therapy, but nothing seemed to work. It just got worse.

At this point in my life, I'd been married three times before Tommy. Each relationship started off on the right foot. The men were impressed with me. Then, slowly my strong personality grated against them, and I would have to lose myself to keep them. I pushed myself inward, and the stress of denying my own essence turned toxic.

That was when the car wreck that led me to yoga left me in persistent, chronic pain—I couldn't move and would be totally dependent on them. *Right where they want me to be*, I'd think. The yoga eventually saved me, but in times of immense stress that pain would flare up and I would resort to opioids. Then the opioids would lead me back to drinking again. As the pain got deeper, my addiction grew stronger.

It was a vicious cycle. I had to have control over something. So using drugs and alcohol was my way to keep control, *I thought.*

All the men in my life enabled me—just like Momma did. They needed me, and I needed them. I chose this type of relationship without even realizing it—to keep the dynamic of the addiction going.

Inevitably, the relationships would end because I could not be myself. I would finally get the courage to be me again and start looking for "Mr. Right." But every single time I thought I found him, our story would turn into a tragedy—*'til I got right with me and God.*

Until this day, being true to myself is still the ultimate challenge.

As tragic as the endings were in my previous marriages, I always felt relief when the ink dried on our divorce papers.

But not with Tommy.

Leaving him left me feeling like half a person. *It was not supposed to be like this.* Tommy and I were supposed to spend our lives together. *Why was this happening?* He felt that way too. He was crushed.

I didn't want to divorce him, but we were too far gone. The final straw came at the end of our very strained marriage, the day he erupted in rage in our bedroom. He beat the closet door off its hinges and tore it to shreds. It scared the living daylights out of me. I had never seen him react like this. At that moment, I began to have flashbacks of all the violence that happened in my childhood home when my daddy would abruptly break into throwing plates across the room, crashing his fist through sheet rock, and knocking my mom across the floor.

I couldn't even recognize Tommy. He had never done anything like this before. I thought, *Oh my God, my husband has become my daddy, and I'm next.*

He was at his wits end—and he used his bare hands to rip apart the door and throw the shreds in every direction in a frenzy of anger. I looked at the pile of splinters and wood—remnants of our closet door, and our marriage, torn to pieces never to be put together again.

Then silence.

I looked with a blank stare and coldly said, "I'm leaving."

I wasn't about to end up married to my daddy.

I moved in with my sponsor at the time, JoAnn. We divorced shortly after, despite the pages and pages of love letters he wrote me pouring out his heart and soul. I had never heard him talk like this, processing his emotions on the page. *All of it.*

I read every line, but I couldn't take them in, or begin to feel empathy toward him, because I was trying so hard to process my own emotions.

The shame I felt about wrecking our future and our dreams—all the things I had done when I was drunk, all the sleepless nights he endured waiting for me while I was blacked out somewhere—it was just too much for me to bear. I couldn't reconcile all that and stay married.

The memories of the shredded door drove me further away.

## Rebuilding the Door

I thought the marriage was over—never to be put back together again. But you know, you can never rely on the way things look, because with God all things are possible. God was about to take the door that Tommy shredded and build us a new one to walk through together. A door that could never be shattered, and could even withstand me going vegan on a Texas cattle ranch!

It was about fourteen years later when Tommy came back into my life. The details are foggy, but here's how Momma tells it. Tommy had a bunch of old-timey VHS tape cassettes that were left over from when we were married. Momma always loved those tapes. Tommy had them all safely stored away and invited her to his house to get the ones she wanted.

As she was packing up the VHS tapes, the two made some conversation.

"Well how are you doing," Mom asked Tommy.

"Fine," he said.

"You got a girlfriend yet," Mom asked flat out.

"I haven't found anyone I care about as much as I love Renée," he said sheepishly.

If memory serves, I called him the next day.

I was selling real estate and making six figures a year. I'd recently divorced my fifth husband and felt confident in the "Renée" I had become. I was sober at the time and it was very attractive to him. I'm sure my three-piece suits, high-heeled shoes, and accessories helped too.

We couldn't agree on where to live—but we knew it had to be together.

By 2009, we had moved in together, and we married again in 2010.

In 2002, he'd acquired a ninety-six-acre, small cattle ranch in Angleton, Texas, and was just a couple of years away from retiring at Dow Chemical. He had picked up the ranching baton of his forefathers and stepped into it as if born to do it. I wasn't keen on walking in high heels through the dirt. I didn't like opening gates. I detested all the bugs and wanted nothing to do with anything remotely resembling cattle ranching. I wanted him to move to Pearland, where I was selling houses and making a killing, but he wouldn't have it.

Tommy was resolute. I thought he was crazy. I felt like I had been catapulted into *Green Acres*, where Zsa Zsa Gabor and her farmer husband have a standoff and eventually, the city girl moves to the country. I always fancied myself a rhinestone cowgirl of sorts, never the muddy, fence-mending, hay-baling type. I did like the idea of having animals around, though.

All I knew was that we had a second chance, and if you're lucky enough to get one of those, you gotta take it.

Tommy and I didn't know it, but we were about to be in the business of second chances.

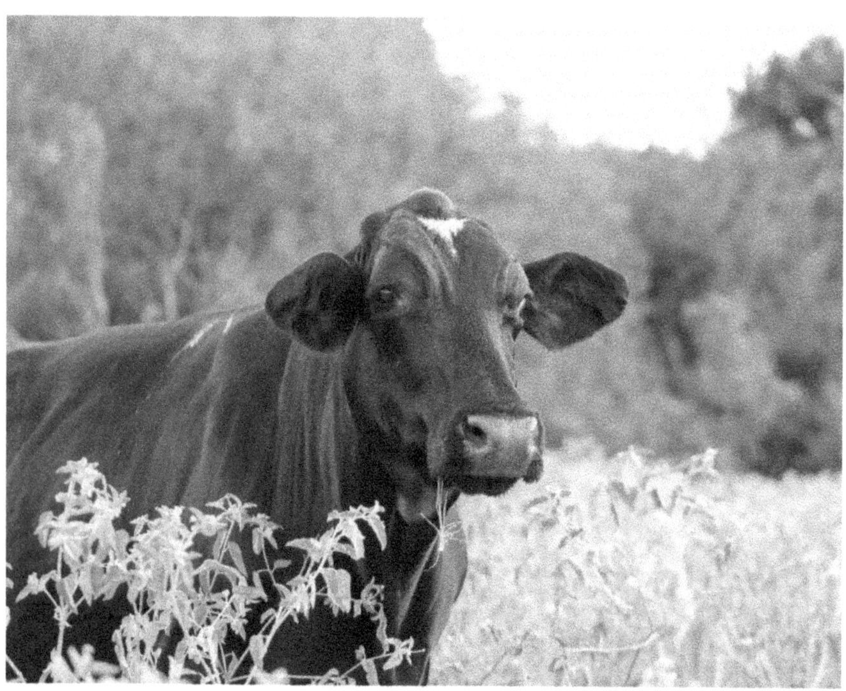

**Figure 4 Rowdy Girl.** *The cow I bottle-fed as a baby, who taught me that love is a covenant I could never again break. She changed my vows, my life, and my destiny.*

# 8

# *Rowdy Girl*

*Rowdy Girl is the cow I bottle fed as a baby—I will most likely name the sanctuary after her! How does that sound? Rowdy Girl Sanctuary!*

*January 3, 2015*

Rowdy Girl is a cow. When people meet me, most think *I'm* Rowdy Girl. I've certainly done enough over the years to earn that reputation. Rowdy Girl changed my entire perception of life, death, families, religion, and food. Without her, I wouldn't be vegan. I might not even be here at all.

I met Rowdy Girl in 2010, the year Tommy and I married for the second time. He came home to tell me about two calves needing a momma up the road, which piqued my interest. I wasn't happy on the ranch. Nothing he did could get me interested in helping him work the cattle, the land, or mending fences. And when I say nothing, I mean *nothing*! I wanted no part of it. That was his bailiwick, and as long as he kept me out of it, I was happy to keep my distance. That was until I heard the words, "Babies needing a momma."

Oh, my goodness, he knew how to pluck my heartstrings.

I tried having a baby for years, but I was sterile. I yearned for the experience of having a child with Tommy, but it was not meant to be. I tried to hang on to my female organs, because I was desperate to have a child—but almost every time I had a period I would land in the ER. The pain was unbearable.

I had an emergency DNC to remove a grapefruit-sized cyst on my ovary that burst and left me riddled with scar tissue.

Eventually, I was diagnosed with endometriosis and found out my fallopian tubes were deformed. To this day, I believe those deformities were created when my momma endured multiple beatings while pregnant with me.

That's when the reality of it hit me hard. The OB-GYN told me I needed a total hysterectomy. I would never have a child of my own.

I was never quite the same after they removed my reproductive organs. I almost died after the operation when I started hemorrhaging in the middle of the night. My blood pressure dropped to 40/20, and they almost lost me. I awoke to a blood transfusion, depressed, and defeated.

Determined to be a momma, I began to search for ways to obtain a surrogate. I pored over websites and ordered materials. They could use Tommy's sperm, carry our baby, and then I'd have my wish. Or maybe we could adopt. I delved into research and explored all the options, but Tommy was never on board, no matter how much I tried to convince him. We fought all the time about the cost and the idea of it all. It wasn't in the cards, and my yearning for a baby was not budging him one bit.

But then, God gave me the baby I was meant to have.

Tommy got the call about two orphaned calves and easily convinced me to go with him to check them out. They were destined to have a momma, and I was destined to be one. They needed me, and I needed them.

He told me they'd need to be bottle-fed, and we could get them for three hundred dollars each, a steal in cattle country. I couldn't wait.

The moment we got there, a bouncy black calf with a white heart on her head came frolicking in my direction. I laughed out loud.

The first words out of my mouth were, "Well, aren't you a little rowdy girl!" That name stuck, and the legend of Rowdy Girl, was christened that day.

The other calf, Bo-Bo (God rest her soul), was not rambunctious at all. She was kind of sickly, but I bought her anyway, along with my Rowdy Girl. Bo-Bo never thrived and died very young, but Rowdy Girl flourished at our ranch, and my relationship with her grew powerfully over the next nine months.

Before Rowdy Girl came into my life, I never woke up wanting to rush outside at dawn to talk to the cows. The day Rowdy Girl came home, I was hooked. She was my child. I didn't want to leave her side. I knew nothing about bottle feeding a calf, so Tommy started teaching me how to mix the formula just right for the babies. He was good at it.

It didn't take me long to figure out how to be a momma. I would rush outside with her "baba" (baby bottle), and as soon as I got to the fence, I would yell, "Rowwwww-dy. Come and get it."

The moment she heard my voice, she would come bouncing and kicking to greet me. The feeling of nourishing a sweet soul that depended solely on me for her well-being is a feeling I cannot describe in any other way than "motherhood." I didn't care if people might find it over the top. I didn't see the difference. She was a child who needed me, and I bonded with her as if she were my own.

As the days grew into weeks, I was drawn deeply into Rowdy Girl's world. While feeding her, she fed me through an etheric umbilical cord that reached into the life force of every bovine in our pasture and beyond.

Something was happening. A miracle was at work. All I knew was that when I was feeding her, she was projecting onto me the sentience of her kind. It was like I was plugged into a cow's DNA while feeding her. In fact, while writing this chapter, I can plug into Rowdy Girl right now and see, feel, and understand bovine language just like humans learn foreign languages.

She was and is my conduit to understanding the plight of cows everywhere. I can feel their pain in my soul. The brutality we inflict on the bovine species and other farmed animals is a blatant act of immense cruelty that damages the psyche of humanity. It has caused violence on our planet to be normalized. Killing them is killing something sacred in us. Rowdy Girl has taught me that if we respect all life, all life will respect us. If we disrespect some lives while honoring others, we will be handed a hell of a karmic blow and there is no getting around it. I wasn't ready for this message.

## My Gift of Desperation

Alcoholism is such a cunning disease.

I had dropped my AA group for a fifth level Reiki practitioner who lived in New York. She told me I was cured of all the past alcoholism and addiction.

She would repeat: "That was Renée then, and this is Renée now." She convinced me I *could* drink. Well, that was music to my alcoholic brain. I thought I was cured of alcoholism.

I went to the grocery store and bought two bottles of expensive Chardonnay and poured myself a glass.

Tommy walked into the room and said, "Renée what are you doing? You can't drink!"

He called my mother, who then called me.

"That was Renée then, and this is Renée now," I told her confidently. "I am cured! Y'all don't have to worry!"

Then I proceeded to drink the entire two bottles. I was on the road to my final desperation. Soon I was drinking every day.

"Renée I need to be able to count on you," Tommy said one afternoon shortly after I had started drinking again. "Can you meet me at the car dealership?"

"Sure," I said.

"Are you sure?" he said tentatively.

"Tommy, I promise I'll be there," I said convincingly. "You can count on me."

Next thing I knew, I went to a bar and blacked out. Cops were called, and I woke up in the emergency room. I was flailing my arms, cursing the doctors.

I touched my hairline and winced. The doctors had put eight or nine stitches in my head.

You would have thought that this incident would have been enough to get me to quit drinking and to debunk the idea that Reiki could cure my alcoholism. *It did not.* In the Alcoholics Anonymous "Big Book," it says you have to be thoroughly convinced of your alcoholism. Even that experience didn't convince me.

Along with alcohol, I was using strong pain medication. The pain in my body was so extreme, but the lingering emotional pain ran way deeper. A pain management specialist gave me thirty vials of Demerol per month, 100 milligrams each. I was prescribed to give myself one injection a day—(as needed for pain). I rarely used only one vial.

Then one day, I used all thirty vials spread out throughout the day. *A thousand milligrams.* I stayed in a Demerol stupor all day, and then passed out on my couch—nearly overdosing.

When I came to, I was drooling and could hardly breathe. I could hear the television. There were familiar phrases from AA coming out of the TV. *Where was I?*

Bill O'Reilly was interviewing two people who were recovering addicts. Christopher Kennedy Lawford and former Congressman Patrick Kennedy shared their experiences on air.

O'Reilly asked, "Can you think of a time where you said, 'Look, I don't want to do this anymore. This is wrecking my body.'"

"Absolutely," Lawford responded. "It wrecks the body. It wrecks the social, you know, relationships with people. I was fairly functional. I went to law school, college, and I got a master certification. But the point was, the disease is really difficult, you have to change everything in your life."

O'Reilly asked, "You couldn't stop."

"I could stop for a little while, and then I'd use again."

My ears perked up. It was like they were talking directly to me. It was like God put an AA meeting right in my freaking living room after nearly overdosing and dying on my couch.

I was transfixed.

"Mr. Kennedy, you were in the House in a high pressure job," O'Reilly continued.

*That's me* I thought. I was addicted to the pressure as much as the substances.

"If you're an addict, you manage your life by consuming drugs and alcohol and managing stress," Kennedy said.

*This is unreal. Is this a dream?* I thought.

"I was drinking at 13." I heard the voices say, and thought, *I started drinking consciously at 14.*

"Were you trying to deaden some pain or something in you?" O'Reilly asked.

*I sure did. I wanted to feel nothing physically, emotionally, mentally, or spiritually. I was like a walking zombie, alive on the outside, but dead on the inside. I was addicted to not feeling my emotions.*

I watched that TV segment over and over again. Then, I went to the bathroom and got all the residual drugs out of the bottles—thinking *maybe I'll use one more time.*

Then I looked in the mirror and didn't see myself. I saw Bill O'Reilly. (I never watched the news or was a particularly big fan), but I couldn't get his image out of my mind. I knew I needed help. The look on my face was like what the Big Book calls the hideous four horsemen: *Terror, bewilderment, frustration, and despair.* I saw them in the mirror.

I had to get help right the f—now.

I called someone.

"Kelly, I need help."

Kelly was a recovering drug user and was someone *I had sponsored* at one point. Without hesitation, she came over and we read some Narcotics Anonymous materials together. Then she took me to an NA meeting.

I walked in the room for the first time as a defeated drug addict. I remember wanting to make myself so small in that meeting. The Big Book talks about hiding underneath a heap—that's exactly what I was feeling:

> *Our twisted relations with family and friends and society at large, that many of us have suffered the most. We have been especially stupid and stubborn about them. The primary fact that we are able to recognize is our total inability to form a true partnership with another human being. Our ego mania digs two disastrous, disastrous pitfalls, either we insist upon dominating the people we know, or we depend on them far too much. Always we tried to struggle to the top of the heap or to hide underneath.*

From underneath that heap I said softly for the first time in my life, "My name is Renée and I am an addict."

I'd always said I was an alcoholic, but not an *addict*. But that was the truth. By naming it, I could finally begin to be released of its grip, and quit lying to myself.

That was January 8, 2013. The day I got clean and sober and my entire worldview and purpose came into focus.

The next day, I called my doctor. My heart was beating out of my chest when I asked the front desk to put me on the phone with him.

"Doctor—my sponsor has told me to call and tell you I am a drug addict. You cannot prescribe me pain medication, and I will not be back to see you," I said.

"Are you sure you don't want to come back to get some medication that is not addicting?" he asked.

"No, I can't do that," I said with finality.

He wished me well, and we hung up the phone.

The pain management doctor was like the grim reaper, and for the first time in my life, I had slammed a steel door in his face. Now, I had to learn how to live and feel without drugs.

The Big Book says, "We in turn sought the same escape with all the desperation of drowning men," and for the first time, I understood what that meant. I was a drowning woman, trapped in the ocean of alcoholism and drug addiction. My way out was complete and total surrender. I reached my hand out of the ocean of alcoholism. God and the program met me there. I had experienced the true gift of desperation. Thank God!

## New Pastures

I began to live by the principle: *to thine own self be true.* That's not easy for someone who has never paused to look at themselves—really look at herself—in the mirror. I was so many things for so many people. I had stuffed my pain down deep. Finally, I could ask myself—*why is Renée here? What purpose did God give her? Why was I spared on my couch that night? Why did I wake up to an AA meeting on my television and land in NA and not in a morgue with a tag on my foot?*

I did all these big, glorious things in my life. I was Miss Renée, the larger-than-life director masquerading as me. It was like I was portraying who I thought I should be. After I got sober I could see clearly for the first time. Like a kaleidoscope coming into focus, I could see how *God* must see me. Things were coming into focus one little slide at a time.

I asked my former sponsor, Sue, if she would sponsor me again. All the years she had known me I was defiant. *I had a really bad case of uniqueness.* She saw me, cycle in and out of the rooms.

Sue had no problem telling me straight up, just like a dirty strong Stoli martini, "You have to find a sponsor *You will obey! do you hear me?"* she hollered.

I had a moment of pause, and then said, "I'll do whatever you say."

"If what I tell you to do works half the time, then it will be better than what you've been doing," Sue said plainly.

That's what hit me between the eyes. This had to be the better way.

The first thing Sue told me was that I needed to take a year off from work to focus on my sobriety. I needed to literally reset my mind and body. It was life or death.

Tommy wasn't thrilled about me not working, but Sue put it to him in cold, hard facts: "Do you want her sober, or do you want her dead?"

It was an obvious answer.

So for the next year, I invested in my sobriety—going to meetings and soaking up AA and NA literature. I would literally write out the Big Book, then record myself reading it, and then listen to myself reading it. *Over and over.*

I wanted to embody the principles and the directions of how to get sober, stay sober, and help others.

After a year, I went to work at the Boys and Girls Club. I did other jobs too. I began selling a supplement called Zeal and making money. I'd play music and tell my story about transformation, and make some sales here and there. Money wasn't the goal at the time, though; focusing on getting rid of all the substances I had put in my body was my aim. All the while I was searching for Renée and learning how to live free from alcohol and drugs for the very first time in my life.

At that time, I wanted to help Tommy more with the ranch. I started paying closer attention to how he ran things and what was going on in our pastures. As people who owned cattle, I thought we should be particular about the milk we drank. *We should get it directly from a milkman*, I thought.

We found a local dairy supplier and were surprised when the deliveries came to our door with the names of the cows on our bottles. It made me feel so good about our choices—drinking Judy's milk, Bonnie's milk, or Della's milk always made me feel justified that we were doing the right thing. It all felt so wholesome.

Next, I thought—OK, we should have our own chickens. *Any good rancher has some chickens.* So we bought some chickens.

Then, I thought, well heck—if we really are ranchers, we should kill one of our own cows and serve the community.

I looked out at the pasture and thought—*which one?* Rowdy Girl had a baby named "Broke Leg." He earned his name after jumping off the trailer when Tommy tried to load him up to go to the sale barn. He walked with a bad limp.

"He won't make it very long," Tommy told me.

Broke Leg was the obvious choice to go to slaughter.

I tried to find other people from the community who would want to go in with us to slaughter Broke Leg.

That's when I started learning more about what we cattle ranchers were really doing with our cows. I started asking Tommy about the process.

He said cows have "one bad day."

*The day they get their throats slit.*

After I started scrutinizing the whole process, I paused and asked myself:

> *What about when they get loaded up in the red trailer? What about when they're separated from their mothers? What about when the mothers cry for days? What about when the babies are dumped off at the sale barn looking with big tearful eyes at the only people they know—betrayed and left behind in total chaos. What about when they get prodded, poked, and pushed around and finally sold to the highest bidder? God only knows what happens to them next.*

The only thing that I knew for certain was that their lives would be filled with suffering until the day they died. All of the things that happen in that process add up to a bunch of bad days. A lot more than one. The way I saw it—our cows suffered immensely from the time they left our pastures to the day they died. By the time their throats were slit, it almost felt like a mercy killing.

You think a cattle rancher's wife thinks, "Hmmm. I think I'll go vegan today." Hell no! I wasn't a vegan. I was just asking questions.

## Rowdy Revolt

It's hard to explain, but I know Rowdy Girl started this revolution in me. I think my final relapse was a way of numbing out the reality of our work as cattle ranchers. I could not look at the pain and suffering of animals when I couldn't even acknowledge my own pain. Now, with a clear mind, I could aim my lifelong defiance at the cattle ranching industry.

When I started loving her like a daughter, I began to reclaim a part of myself—a part that was probably burned in another lifetime. Long-forgotten memories began to surface as I realized Rowdy Girl was like my child. How could I feel this intensity of emotion for a calf? Loving her—and following my heart—opened a hidden door in my soul. It brought me back to myself… and to my purpose.

It was like an ethical uprising, surging from the base of my heart. I didn't know I was going vegan at the time—but I was. I was becoming a key witness to a taboo relationship. Rowdy Girl didn't just make me a mother; my love for her and her kin turned me into a witness—and once I saw the truth, the revolt was inevitable.

Waking up—seeing all of this through Rowdy Girl—gave me a front-row seat to the truth behind animal agriculture. Suddenly, I wasn't just living on a ranch. I was living inside the story that billions of animals endure every single day.

Once I saw the truth, it was like waking up inside the Matrix. I couldn't stay silent—not when I could never unsee the reality of their suffering or the way we were contributing to it every single day through our cow/calf operation. And guess who's doing the talking? Rowdy Girl—through me. Our voices have become one resounding message. I'm in the front row every second of the day. And together, we are on the frontlines of defiance.

But the truth is, it's hard to watch. Once you're there, you can't look away. Rowdy Girl didn't just wake me up—she made me a threat to Big Ag. Just by loving her, I crossed a line I could never uncross. That's why we have to unplug from the machine. There has to be a Rowdy Revolt.

# 9

# *Big Ag: The Three-Headed Snake*

In the beginning of time, there was no "Big Ag." Ten thousand years ago, humanity shifted from foraging to farming. That's when we started domesticating animals for labor—transportation, skins, milk, and cheese. We used goats in the mountains and cattle on ranches, all based on survival.

What began as survival back then evolved into an entire empire of exploitation—a global monstrosity that exploits animals on every scale.

Animal agriculture is an ingredient in our way of life. It's baked into our traditions, our holidays, our economy. Everyone grows up thinking it's normal and necessary.

We've built concentrated feedlots—hellholes pumped with antibiotics and violence. A hellhole we created right here on Earth.

We slaughter over eighty to ninety billion land animals every year. Most of them are babies—chickens at just six weeks old, pigs at six months, cows before their second birthday. They never get to grow up. They never get to live natural lives. Their childhood is stolen in the name of food, profit, and tradition. This is the truth we hide behind cellophane packages and barbecue sauce. But once you see it, you can't unsee it. And once you feel it—really feel it—you can't ever go back.

Animal agriculture is worth an estimated $1.6–$3.3 trillion dollars per year. We colonized the land—land that belonged to everyone—including the animals. We monopolized the food systems, and with that, our politics. We are in a death grip. Revolutionizing animal agriculture automatically revolutionizes our government. It's that huge.

It's not an industry. It's an institution.

## Dominion and Abusive Systems

The meat industry mirrors every abusive structure I've ever survived. It doesn't just create dominance—it amplifies it. And it's hard to see, because living inside of it is like walking through one of those carnival mirror mazes. Everything's distorted. You can't tell what's real. You think it's normal—until you find your way out.

Using the backs of animals, they control the very land people live on. They dominate their movements, confining them to hellish conditions. They control their reproduction, their babies, and their bodies.

We took them out of the wild and turned them into food. It's like Soylent Green—but instead of people, it's animals. Mothers and their babies. Lives with bonds and feelings, reduced to flesh on a plate. Eating flesh has been normalized, wrapped in myth, defended by tradition, and justified with religion. And the real kicker? It wasn't just brute force. It was a blessing at the table of family gatherings. They used religion to dress it up in disgusting holiness. They made it sanctimonious and it's sickening.

We were told humans were made in God's image—and that animals were made for us. When God said, "I give you charge over the animals," or "to name them," we twisted it. We turned caretaking into control. Dominion into domination.

And that domination didn't stop with animals. It's the same thread that runs through how we've treated women, other races, other nations—anyone we wanted to conquer, by God! Big Ag perfected the system. They built a business model on exploitation and motherhood—on the backs of those who scream behind slaughterhouse walls, the vulnerable, and the ones we pretend not to see.

## Women Healers

Since the dawn of time, the moment humans learned to control animals and their reproduction, that same control was turned on those who embodied nature, nurtured life, and served as the original caretakers—women. That ain't no coincidence. We were the ones who understood the rhythms of the Earth—and they couldn't stand that kind of power living beyond their control.

We were the good stewards of the land and the animals. It's known that women were the keepers of the rhythms of life. Women worked with nature, not against it. We used our intuition to heal—with food, herbs, and touch. We honored the seasons. We were called witches. Not because we were evil—but because we were free. The ones who experience true freedom are always exploited.

We burned women at the stake so that Big Pharma could own the herbs. So long as women didn't have a soul, we could control them. So long as animals were considered soulless, we could exploit them.

## Three-Headed Snake

When I think about patriarchy, I see how they've made God into an angry and warring masculine force. To believe that God is only masculine is insanity—a father figure only? *Where's Mom?* That belief has become so deeply perverted.

When women started pushing back against that system, they were burned alive—for doing what modern medicine is still trying to understand. If we could access that natural energy, we would remember how to take care of the earth, the animals, the environment, and each other.

And what came after? Science. Big Science. Big Intellect. Not to make us free—but to control our bodies with pharmaceuticals and medical procedures.

That's when Big Pharma and Big Medicine were born. The wisdom of the herbalists, midwives, and healers was dismissed—and replaced with pills, scalpels, and sterile white coats. We used to heal with our hands, with food, with fasting, with presence. But they pathologized the body, dissected it, and monetized natural healing. They turned healing into a business. They made us afraid of our own intuition, our own rhythms—our own power.

What should have been a prescription for living was sterilized and sold back to us as treatment—we were cut off from nature, spirit, and the breath of life itself. And it hurt us. The remedies they sold us didn't just wound us—they beat us into submission with false hope. They betrayed the body, broke trust with the Earth, left us starving for wholeness, and convinced us we were healed.

Everything was designed that way. It stopped being about holistic healing and became all about selling—selling the ads, the procedures, the pills, the lies. If we were really free, we wouldn't have to fight so hard to live, to eat good food, and to drink good water. Food became a product, not a birthright.

We should've been taught how to grow our own food, how to trust the land and our own hands. Instead, we are sold processed junk laced with GMOs—foods that feed the very sicknesses that make us dependent on Big Pharma and Big Medicine.

They're all in bed together. It's like the devil himself: Big Ag, Big Pharma/Medicine, and Big Religion—a three-headed snake. Each one depends on keeping us disconnected from our bodies, our instincts, and the truth.

And it all goes back to the same lie: Dominion. The myth that dominion keeps you safe and that it's righteous.

But real safety was never about control—it was always about connection and community.

## Factory Farming

When we think of factories, we picture machines—assembling shoes, tables, and stuff like that. But on a farm—especially a factory farm—you're not just producing a "so called" product. You're manufacturing misery in extreme proportions. It's the dark underbelly of our food system. A mechanized beast that devours life void of empathy.

As my friend and leading animal rights activist Jamie Logan says: "We are so disconnected from the individuals behind the price tag, it allows us to comply, exploit them, and not see them for the individuals that they are."

Life gets processed—stripped down, packaged, and sold—like a shoelace, long before it ever reaches the final product.

That's what woke me up.

We were sending our animals into that killing machine. Every animal who enters that machine will experience extreme violence with no mercy.

To be born into the world of animal agriculture, for example, on a dairy farm, means this:

A calf is taken from her mother within hours of birth.

If it's a male, he might starve in a crate, be shot in the head, or be sold for veal.

If it's a female, she'll be forced into the same cycle as her mom—impregnated again and again, her babies taken each time. And instead of nursing her own, she'll be hooked up to machines and milked for humans until their bodies completely give out.

Her milk—meant for her babies—will never reach them. Instead, she will grieve her losses time and time again. And nobody comes to her rescue.

And her body will be used up and give out long before her natural life is over.

In the case of a piglet, it might suckle for a short while—but not with her mother free to nurture her. Soon, she's crammed into metal pens with concrete floors, packed in with others without sunlight or fresh air. No dirt to root in, no grass to play on and no relief in sight—just endless torture and confinement living life in a bed of feces and urine. Their tails are cut off—either sliced with a blade or burned off, and their teeth are clipped with pliers or ground down to the gum line. And if any of those piglets are too weak to live, they are dashed to death on the floor.

For male piglets? Their scrotum is sliced open with a sharp blade, and then their testicles are yanked off without anesthesia. They scream and writhe and often go into shock.

The "lucky" females will spend a lifetime in forced confinement, impregnated again and again and locked into a gestation crate so small she can't even turn around. Once she gives birth, she'll be moved to a farrowing crate, where her babies can nurse, but she still can't even turn around. Oftentimes, they go crazy just trying to move.

Her body will eventually give out after three or five years—after a constant cycle of suffering. She'll be bruised and broken before she's finally sent to slaughter.

The screaming never stops.

The urine, the feces, the blood, the guts—where does it all go?

It doesn't just disappear. It runs off into our water, seeps into our soil, and pollutes the air and our bodies.

The suffering doesn't stay inside the factory—it spills out into the world.

And we breathe it. We drink it. We live in it.

The violence we do to them doesn't stay hidden. It always finds its way back to us. And some of the most fragile animals, like chickens, endure the worst of it. Egg-laying hens are stacked in warehouse cages, barely able to move. Some go mad, breaking their own legs and pulling off their own feet in the metal cages trying to escape.

And the babies? The little male chicks are ground up alive in hatcheries—no use for boys in the egg industry.

Those raised for meat are genetically engineered to grow too big and too fast—their bodies ballooning with unnatural muscle in just a few weeks.

They collapse under their own weight and are slaughtered at six or seven weeks old.

I call them Franken-chickens. They're designed for profit, not for life. Just like those cows you see on the side of the road in "peaceful" pastoral settings—there's always suffering behind the illusion.

Cows raised for beef are ear-tagged and branded young.

They spend time with their momma, bond with her, nurse from her—and then are torn away around six months old when they're rounded up and sold at auction. This causes extreme trauma and stress for both the momma and the baby.

At auction, a few bulls and heifers will be bought as breeding stock, but most will go to a feedlot. There they will endure the next stage of their suffering before being slaughtered. The older or "spent" animals will go directly to their death.

On the feedlot, they'll be fattened up in an overcrowded trough where they'll stand knee-deep in feces. They'll be pumped full of antibiotics just to survive the filth and disease. And then they'll go to slaughter.

On their way to the kill floor, they will hear the screams of those being killed before them. They'll smell the blood. They'll feel pure terror—and again there will be no mercy. No rescue. No coming home. Slaughterhouses are built for speed, not compassion.

No one stops to care that the animals are suffering. Even the workers—often undocumented or formerly incarcerated—are exploited. They're underpaid, overworked, and pushed to their breaking point. Mistakes are common. Throats are slit while eyes are still blinking—because the bolt gun fails. Some are dismembered while still alive. It is a complete nightmare.

And this isn't just happening in some faraway third-world country. It's happening right here in our hometowns—*Legally*. It's masterfully and intentionally hidden in plain sight—with rolling hills and picturesque pastures hiding the horror of animal agriculture.

But if you see it—*really see it*—a Rowdy Girl is born.

# 10

# *The Moment I Went Vegan*

*Hey Y'all! Happy Halloween. And more importantly, Happy Vegan Birthday to me! This was truly a spooky day for me. Honestly, it continues to reverberate with spooky feelings into the present. It's appropriate in a way that it was on Halloween, when it is said that the veil between the spirit and the corporeal world thins.*

*October 31, 2022*

It was Halloween 2014, and I had been watching slaughterhouse videos all morning. I didn't know I was going down the vegan rabbit hole. I had tried to take some of this information in, before I relapsed, but it was too much for me. The realities of what I kept stumbling on were too painful for me to process. I was in denial. I didn't want to feel anything, so I would use drugs and alcohol. But now sober, I was facing my feelings and the consequences of what that meant head on.

*Who had I become? A cattle rancher's wife—signing off on all of this killing?*

In researching what happens to cows when they leave our pastures, I landed on horrific slaughterhouse videos day after day... *for months.*

I was in shock and I was obsessed. I walked around carrying the weight of their pain, and it matched my own.

My eyes were constantly red and puffy. I would sob uncontrollably night after night while Tommy was in the next room, trying to watch the news.

For the first time, the pain and agony that I had never been able to express was meeting me in the suffering of the animals. I felt their suffering like it was my own.

Time and time again, I'd wail in agony like a mother cow losing her babies.

Poor Tommy would just turn up the TV, and occasionally holler at me to stop watching those "goddamn PETA propaganda videos."

I remembered back to my early-twenties—back when that pastor threatened me after I witnessed him sexually abusing his children. "If you tell anyone what you saw, I'll put you through a meat grinder, and no one will ever know what happened to you."

Those words echoed in my body: *A meat grinder. Like an animal's body put through a meat grinder. Like my animals.* I remember the helplessness I felt in that moment—with no one advocating for me. I was terrified.

Now sober, it was like their pain was a mirror of my own suffering.

Again, I wasn't a vegan at this point in my life, but I was having feelings that were in direct opposition to the way I should be feeling as a cattle rancher's wife. I could not stuff these feelings down anymore—knowing full well that if I did, *I would use*. I was either going to go crazy and die or save the cows.

On this particular day, I was being pulled into the land of the living. I was leaving my old life behind, and I didn't know it. I was shedding the old and getting ready for the new. All I knew was that my heart was breaking, my soul was shattering, and my mind was exploding, trying to comprehend the other side—the side where animals are friends, not food.

During this awakening, I stumbled upon Melanie Joy's dissertation on carnism (an invisible belief system or ideology that conditions people to eat certain animals). I was a wreck. We had plans to be at Effie's house (Tommy's mother) that afternoon, and I had to get my shit together.

*Just one more video*, I reasoned. Something that might educate me a little instead of tormenting me with images of sadness, despair, and lots of blood.

I hit play and proceeded to watch a family sitting at the kitchen table having dinner. I remember there was a fresh tablecloth, and everyone was waiting to be served by the lady of the house. The main course was beef stew.

The conversation heightened as the lady of the house ladled the steaming hot stew into their bowls. Everyone was savoring the deliciousness of the beef stew.

Finally, someone said, "This is delicious. What's the recipe?"

The lady of the house said, "Well, you start off with a pound of very young golden retriever." Everyone stopped eating with their mouth wide open in disbelief. No one could continue their meal. They seemed suspended in time.

Now I know that they were in that *in-between place* where the veil is pierced and a moment of clarity is dawning.

That moment of clarity hit them square in the face, the way it did me.

I remember it to this day because I was with them on the other side of the screen. My mouth flew open in horror, and I instantly realized that I could be eating *anybody's* body. It could be a dog, a cat, or even a person, and I wouldn't even know it, because the meat would be hacked up into tiny pieces of flesh.

*Good God,* I thought.

At that moment, while watching the video in slow motion, the lady of the house said: "Just kidding, it's really a cow."

I was so upset, and so were the folks dining at the table on the computer screen. They could not continue with their lunch. The image of a puppy chopped to bits was now front and center in their consciousness. Try as they might, they could not bring themselves to eat the rest of the beef stew. They set their utensils down.

I began to sob. *Again*!

Tommy was fed up. At that moment, he reminded me with great disgust that we had somewhere to be and that I needed to pull myself together.

I shook the memory of that scene off, washed my face, put on my makeup, and got dressed. With that, we were off to the yearly Halloween block party at Effie's house.

I didn't know that I was gonna go vegan that day.

No vegans held flags, shouted, or fell over in the street protesting with blood on their bodies. There was just the unrelenting torture of my own soul, searing through the veil of cultural conditioning, traditional programming, and religious upbringing.

On this day, I had trouble crossing over from this new paradigm, where animals were friends and not food. How could I go back to filling the role of "good rancher's wife"? I had one foot down the rabbit hole and the other on this godforsaken Earth that made no sense to me.

*"Which way do I go, which way do I go?"*

The words kept ringing in my soul.

I didn't know I was going vegan, but Rowdy Girl did. I really do believe that she was the master conductor in all of it.

We walked into Effie's house on Mesquite Street in Lake Jackson, Texas. The living room was buzzing with laughter, conversation, and Halloween charm.

All of a sudden, I felt like I was in a horror movie. All the kids wore their costumes, and the smell of dead bodies wafted through the air. My stomach turned. Everything moved in slow motion. I was sober, so I knew I wasn't hallucinating, but I felt weirdly disconnected. I could hear, see, and smell, but my senses were acute. The wind in the air was right that day, just like it was when I met Tommy.

That's when the vegan genie came out to play, and just like that, I was snatched down the rabbit hole.

"Renée," said my mother-in-law, "Would you like a bowl of beef stew?"

Her words sounded like a trumpet over the sounds of family love and communion.

"*No*," I said, "I can't eat *that*."

It was like I already knew the script!

*How could this be? I had just watched this very scene play out on my computer screen!*

It was like when the actors come out of the screen in the movie *The Purple Rose of Cairo.*

*What the hell was going on? Am I in a movie?*

"Well, why not, Renée?" My mother-in-law asked.

Before I could think, the truth flew out of my mouth for the first time in my life.

I called it out at the table in front of God and everybody.

"Because it's got floating hacked-up dead animal bodies in it, and I can't eat *that*!"

You could've heard a pin drop. Time stood still for everyone, just like in the video I'd just watched an hour before.

Frozen in my memory are mouths wide open, eyes shocked, all pointed at me. Children in costume looked around at the family, wondering what had just happened. Poor Tommy was shaking his head in disbelief.

"Well, Renée, you can pick it out," my mother-in-law said—God rest her soul.

"There's *no* more pickin' it out for *me*," I said to her, as much as to myself, as that moment of clarity dawned on me.

All my life, I've tried to fit into everyone's thoughts and ideas about who I should be and what I should do with my life, particularly when it came to the men I got involved with. Whether I was married to them, working for them, or they were a family member, I always felt a need to please them. I became absorbed in their work and thoughts about how I should act, dress, and so on. However, the chemistry of me plus male energy always sucked the life out of me. I went vegan and instantly felt my power. I was a woman who could do anything. Damn!

A force greater than myself began to surge through my body. It was just like when I got sober. I knew beyond a shadow of a doubt that I would never eat animals again.

No man, woman, mother, daddy, brother, sister, nobody could shake my resolve to see the animals we used to send to slaughter as my friends and family. Everything started falling into place, and it all made sense to me now. I knew the work I was here to do. My spiritual path and my work had finally converged. There was no stopping me now.

I wasn't raised to follow my intuition. I was raised with the idea that marriage was the ultimate goal—that's why I did it six times (twice to Tommy). Culture didn't look kindly on a woman who listened to herself, who bucked tradition and went her own way. I always did it anyway. But that day, I heard my destiny *loud* and *clear*. What an empowering thing it was to find my authentic voice at the bottom of that rabbit hole. I was transfixed by the sound of it, and I had no idea it was about to lead me to a revolution.

I really do believe God used Rowdy Girl, the slaughterhouse videos, and the Melanie Joy video to bring it all together for me on that day, at that time, and at that moment.

We went from Halloween to "War of the Roses" overnight. By God, no more animal products would be consumed in my home. I was playing with fire on a Texas cattle ranch, married to a multigenerational cattle rancher who was madder than a hornet. In the back of his mind and mine was the obvious question. *Did this mean a second divorce? Would my going vegan end my marriage for the second time?*

Whatever the consequences, I was going to do whatever it took to go deeper down that rabbit hole.

What happened next was Tommy's worst nightmare.

# 11

# *'Til Death Do Us Part*

*When I first learned the truth, I tortured myself with hours upon hours of graphic footage of slaughterhouses and animal farms, weeping uncontrollably, as my resolve to end this abuse came together starting at home—no more animal products for me, and eventually no more deer heads on the wall, no more meat-eating husband and no more cattle ranch! Prior to my vegan awakening, I looked away. I had the faintest soul murmurings that this didn't sit right, but I stuffed them away and tried to be a good cattle rancher's wife.*

*March 4, 2025*

Going vegan was likely gonna be the "death of me" and my marriage, but, by golly, I would never allow the cows on our land to go to slaughter again.

It seems my life has always been reminiscent of a scary Halloween story. With a flair for the dramatic, I always seemed to attract the perfect potion of deadly love and extreme behaviors.

The "death of me" never scared me. I'd spent plenty of time on the verge of life and death with an uncanny ability to skate that fatal line. I was hell-bent on challenging death at every turn, mine and anyone else's who dared get too close to me or tried to hurt anyone I loved—just like I tried to kill my daddy when he was trying to kill my momma.

I loved Rowdy Girl, and now her life was on the line.

My entire world was about to change. Every decision I made at that moment took me closer to the brink of no return. I was plunging a knife into my husband's spine. Only this time, it wasn't a butcher's knife. It was my vegan heart. My going vegan killed my husband's pride, and it destroyed that part of my traditional Christian upbringing that had taught me that it was God's will for us to kill and eat animals.

Tommy and I rode home in silence on the way back from Effie's house. The tension between us was palpable. My heart skipped a beat as soon as we entered the driveway to our cattle ranch in Angleton. My entire perception had changed. The day before, it was the Sonnen Ranch full of cows going to slaughter, but the moment I went vegan it was a haven, full of cows that were my family and that would never be food. All the money and resources, and all the folks I knew were gonna line up to support my mission because, by God, it was the right thing to do. In my mind, all of Texas was about to go vegan.

Before I was sober and vegan, I didn't have much regard for life. In an instant, it became my passion. When I got sober, I wanted to live—really live—for the first time. And when I went vegan, I wanted to do everything I could to take care of my cows. Before that they were just black blobs out in the pasture. After I went vegan, they became individuals. I could identify each and every one of them for their unique personalities and physical characteristics.

I could feel Rowdy Girl's heartbeat coursing through my veins. As the truck slowed in the driveway, I looked around with tears flowing down my cheeks. Every feeling I had stuffed within me was now breaking out on the surface of my skin. The vegan in me was roaring, and my mind, heart, and emotions were challenged to keep up with my rebirth.

I walked through the door behind an exhausted Tommy and death gripped me. Our walls were covered in trophies. The dead heads of deer and other wildlife that were always present, at once, overtook me. I ducked my head and frantically rushed to the bedroom to hide. The remorse, regret, and utter disgust I felt for living in a house consumed with relics and treasures representing death was unbearable. A scream of pain burst from the core of my being.

"Tommy," I yelled.

I was frantic.

"We need to have a funeral for all the animals that you killed. Go outside and dig a thirty-foot hole and bury them. They deserve a proper burial and memorial."

The look on his face was rigid and contorted.

"What?" he exclaimed. "You are f–ing crazy!"

"Yes," I yelled. "We've determined that, and I'm never coming back!"

We exploded. It was a wild flurry. We raged and said terrible things to each other. Tommy and I had fought before, but this put every other argument we'd ever had to shame. In the living room of our home, central to the space we occupied every single day, was a huge elk head that his grandfather had killed in 1947. Tommy was so proud of that elk head. He affectionately considered it a family heirloom!

In my mind, I wanted to string Tommy Sonnen up and hang him from the antlers of that elk. I imagined us just like the couple in the movie *War of the Roses*, who battle each other swinging from the chandelier. I imagined Tommy and me fighting to the death over that poor beautiful elk that died only to be remembered as a family heirloom.

My new vegan brain was quickly processing the world around me in a different light. I was filled with shame, sadness, and anger.

*How have we, as a species, ever come to think of animals in this way?* I thought.

On this day, even though I loved Tommy, I hated what he represented—hunting, killing, fishing, and slaughtering. *Death, death, and death.* Death celebrated was the worst! Our outbursts and our sudden hatred for what each of us stood for and against were immense. I loudly called him a murderer, repeatedly blasting him with one tirade after the next in my attempt to make sense of who I had married.

Tommy Sonnen had always been the perfect gentleman. He was kind, soft-spoken, and a lover of animals. We always had a house full of cats, dogs, and even raccoons. But suddenly, my perception of him shifted. The kind-hearted man I had always known and married not once but twice was now a bloodthirsty maniac, hell-bent on defending his right to kill and eat animals.

His defense was all wrapped up in familial loyalty, cultural norms, and traditional values. His many reasons were valid to the rapidly disintegrating carnist part of my brain. The vegan brain would have none of it. There was no reason good enough to justify his participation in the suffering and death of animals. I was going to save them all, every last one.

"Till death do us part" took on new meaning. I knew in my heart that Tommy was a good man. Tommy was a hunter, who believed killing animals for food was righteous. *But I just knew he would choose kindness over killing if I could ever get him to see it.* Tommy's unrelenting right to slaughter animals for food was unflinching, lighting the way forward toward the death of our second marriage, but I made it my business to challenge him on every front, whether family, tradition, or culture.

My methods were not kind in the beginning. I was brutal. But, if you're gonna stay married to a cattle rancher and go vegan, you better get ready to come out swinging and get ready for a vegan rodeo. They really are a thing, and I've come to enjoy the fight as long as I'm on the side of the animal's rights. Nobody can ever tell me again that breeding and killing animals for food is justified.

Old habits, traditions, and normalized violence die hard. The fact that Tommy and I were back together, married for the second time, was a miracle. I was sober, and for the first time in my life, I was taking my sobriety seriously, and asking questions like: *How could God really put our marriage vows in the balance again? Would my going vegan end my second marriage?*

There was no way I would let that happen without a real fight, but Tommy Sonnen didn't stand a chance.

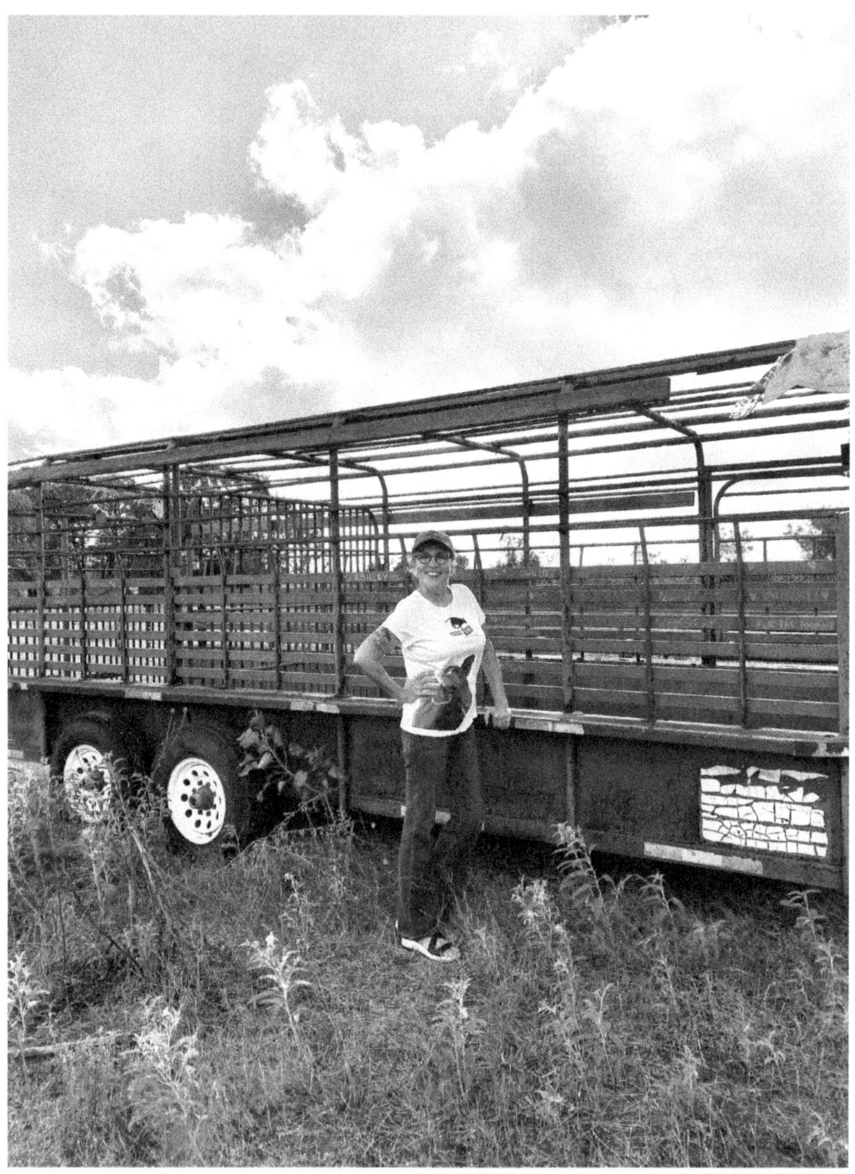

**Figure 5 Red Trailer.** *The red trailer is a symbol of the heartache that I felt each time the babies would be loaded up for auction. The sound of families torn apart tormented me. Now the red trailer is a symbol of hope—it became my promise to them that never again would I betray their trust.*

# 12

# *Becoming a Cowgirl*

*I love cows like family, and they've fired my imagination to go beyond my limited belief systems of normalized cruelty and injustice toward animals. My soul yearns to be in their presence. It is with them that I've learned to be myself instead of the self programmed by society.*

*July 12, 2021*

After my vegan awakening, we slept in separate rooms. Being in the same room with Tommy sickened me. Who was this man? I was married to a killer. *How could I legitimately go from loving someone to despising him overnight?*

I awoke before sunrise, hurriedly dodged the decapitated heads hanging on my walls, and had some breakfast. I chanted the Gayatri mantra, a four-thousand-year-old Sanskrit chant I learned during my yogic spiritual studies. This Vedic prayer is about illumination and calls in divine light—that radiant source of our Creator—(and Lord knows I needed all the light, power, and help I could get at this point).

I said this and *all* my prayers—the Third-Step prayer, the Seventh-Step Prayer, the Eleventh-Step Prayer, the Lord's Prayer, the Serenity Prayer. You name it, I was prayin' it. But that morning, I prayed like I never prayed before, trying to harness heaven as I communed with the cows.

The weather was perfect for a stroll through the cow pasture. It was a bit foggy, and the sun was peeking over the horizon. My senses were sharp. I could see and hear the cows grazing peacefully.

*How did I not see them before? What kind of societal toxin had I been subjected to?*

It was difficult to comprehend my heart space that morning. Every molecule in my body was being reeducated to point zero. My DNA was shuffling as fast as possible to keep up with the new belief system I had triggered. On this very sacred day, I would live out my first twenty-four hours as an ethical vegan. Relishing this day was paramount to my experience.

In the past, I'd been a vegetarian on and off during my yoga and Ayurveda training. I even experienced a raw plant-based diet when I went to the Optimal Health Institute in Austin, Texas, for a two-week cleanse in 2002 to detox from opiates. But this was different. I wasn't "going vegan" because of a decision to feel better, eat better, or educate myself. I was doing it for the animals.

It's a lot like getting sober. You can stop drinking and still be what we call a "dry drunk" if you don't change and aren't willing to go to any lengths to stay sober. You have to have a spiritual awakening that changes everything—or you're probably going to get drunk.

For me, becoming an ethical vegan was parallel to that spiritual awakening I had when I got sober. It was then that I knew that I would never eat any more animals on purpose.

When I became an ethical vegan, I started asking questions regularly—every meal, every restaurant, every trip to the grocery store. My consciousness had become one with the animals. I couldn't make excuses anymore about not knowing *who* I was eating.

I saw and realized the truth: Animals are just like us. They have their own communities, families, and reasons for being here. Their reason for being here is not so they can be food for humans.

*Was my pineal gland finally awakening? Is this what is meant by your kundalini rising?* The truth had always been there. In my kundalini yoga training, I remember learning the phrase *Sat Nam*, which means "truth is my name." In teacher training, we would sit and chant long Sat Nams for eleven minutes every day, along with a host of other chants intended to activate our true yogic nature. The vibration of the ancient Gurmukhi language is said to awaken the truth in you if you practice every day for long periods.

Well, I'm here to tell ya that not only have I chanted long Sat Nams for years, but I've also resonated deeply with Sanskrit and Gurmukhi chanting. There's something about the vibrational cleansing of the sound frequencies that are emitted in the practitioner's body, mind, and soul over time. I woke up on my first day being a vegan and felt a deep calling to chant. It was a true awakening on every level.

I'd heard for years that when you practice the ancient teachings of yoga, you *become* yoga over time. The trappings of conditioning gradually leave you, and what emerges is the truth of who you truly are. The truth of who you came to be in this life emerges. I could feel myself becoming truer.

I could feel myself yet again, awakening, yet again recovering.

In this space, I went outside, opened the gate, and entered the world of the cows. I was speechless. The sound of blood was rushing into my ears. I distinctly recall my hands on the cold and wet latch and felt I was entering a world more deeply than ever before. Yet I had walked through it begrudgingly many times with Tommy. Side-by-side, on the same land with the same cows, the same girl, and the same guy, an alternate reality existed. Now, for the first time, I felt initiated. I was becoming a true "cowgirl."

I went from a city slicker in leather boots to a bona fide vegan cowgirl that would never consider harming a hair on an animal's head, let alone sell them to be killed. The eyes of all the cows were looking in my direction as if they knew. My breathing slowed to a deliberate *ujjayi* breath—breathing life in, breathing death out—and I began to chant Sat Nam.

Spontaneously, I began to sing *Truth Is My Name*. I started chanting *Om*, which is synonymous with the unborn seed of life itself—the very sound of the universe.

With every step I took, I felt myself going deeper into the heartbeat of what was once a cattle ranch, experiencing my new vegan vibration for the very first time. It was clear to me that this land needed cleansing. A primeval memory of how to do that began. Generations of cattle had grazed this land—cattle raised and bred for slaughter. My yogic spirit was on fire to clear the violent channels of the ninety-six acres that would become the original home of Rowdy Girl Sanctuary.

I didn't know at the time that we would become a sanctuary. I didn't realize we were destined to be the world's first documented beef cattle ranch to care for cows instead of killing them. However, as I took each step into their world, I became them. Every step, breath, and sound I uttered channeled their energy, rights, language, and message. I was their redemption, and they were mine. With every breath, I entered their consciousness with the assurance that I would do whatever was necessary to save them from slaughter. I promised them.

Putting it all in perspective as a human in modern society is impossible. One must part the Red Sea of collective conditioning in order to enter a world where true kindness is normal. We must sit with a simple but hard question.

*How can we love animals and kill them?*

Tears fell from my eyes as I walked through the herd. Deep guttural sounds of grief poured out of me. I groaned for forgiveness. Dropping to my knees in the middle of the herd, I wept uncontrollably. Placing my head and hands on the earth, I imagined the truth of our Heavenly Mother coursing into the top of my crown chakra. With every tear that fell to the ground, I felt her healing my mind of human conditioning.

I had always looked to the sky for our Heavenly Father, but in this moment, I recognized how in step we are with Mother Earth.

> *We were supposed to take care of the Earth and all its inhabitants. We have done the opposite. We are killing our Mother and the animals. Our planet has become a breeding ground for death and suffering.*

Despite the way we treat her, I felt for the first time the love the Earth has *for us.*

The vegan transition coursed through my *ida*, *pingala*, and *sushumna* (yogic terms for the etheric channels that animate us all).[1] With every breath out, I imagined dumping into the dirt my false beliefs about animals being here for us to eat. I buried that concept of our distorted dominion over animals. Mother Earth took it all from me.

My body shook as I was relieved of the violence of every body I had eaten.

I purged everyone, and at the end of the meditative experience, I was spent. I was clean and clear of all the blood and bodies I had drained.

In this space, all my memories began to awaken to the truth. It was tough not to hate my parents, my teachers, the church, and my cattle ranching husband.

Why were we conditioned to eat innocent beings when it was now clear as a bell that animals are here *with* us, not *for* us?

I wanted to scream from the top of my lungs to the universe.

I'll never know the moment when animal blood and flesh first entered my body as food, but I know for a fact that if I had never been fed blood and bodies, I would have never chosen to eat them. I was born vegan but was conditioned to be a vampire instead.

Death becomes us when we eat it. That's plain and simple to me now. The real God of creation never intended His children to eat each other. I truly believe that the God of creation intended all beings, even the carnivores we know today, to be vegan. Eden, according to the Book of Genesis, was vegan:

> "Then God said, "I give you every seed-bearing plant on the face of the whole earth and every tree that has fruit with seed in it. They will be yours for food."
>
> (Genesis 1:29)

In Isaiah 11:6, it says, "And the wolf will dwell with the lamb, and the leopard will lie down with the kid, and the calf and the young lion and the fatling together; and a little boy will lead them."

*If God never intended us to eat each other, is veganism the real blueprint for our planet?* I wondered.

Hosea 2:18 says, "In that day I will make a covenant for them with the beasts of the field, the birds in the sky and the creatures that move along the ground. Bow and sword and battle I will abolish from the land so that all may lie down in safety."

"Mooooooo!" At that moment, I looked up from the ground where my head had been pressing against it in a fetal position. The cows surrounded me. All around me, as close to me as they could get, they enveloped me. I could smell their damp, thick skin, which triggered my olfactory memory, reminding me of the smell of leather. It sickened me. But feeling the warmth of their breath, their eyes penetrating mine, once more I wept uncontrollably. I didn't want to leave their presence. I was them, and they were me. We were one.

Slowly, I stood up. The cows didn't move. Surrounded by my new friends, I raised my arms to the heavens, interlaced my fingers, and pointed my index fingers to pierce the sky and the planetary stars beyond. At the same time, I grounded my feet deliberately into the energy of the earth beneath me and chanted three long Sat Nams, the Gayatri Mantra, and ended with three long Oms.

While chanting, I visualized the death of carnism. I envisioned it leaving my body and falling to the ground like fertilizer. Out of all of the death, the subtle energies of all the suffering would become like a sacred compost for a new beginning.

The awakening of who I truly was fell in a rain from the heavens and into the antenna of my index fingers. The energy was fierce as it spiraled into my seventh chakra[2] and coursed through the channels of my soul. I was becoming the vegan I was always meant to be, the vegan I believe we are all meant to be. Veganism is recovery from carnism. It's more than a dietary decision or a health hack. With intention and openness, veganism can be a spiritual awakening that moves us toward kindness, humility, justice, and even forgiveness.

I lowered my hands, looked deeply into the eyes of each cow in my presence, and began walking through them for the first time as one of them, without fear. They all moved to let me through as my vegan vision quest began.

# 13

# *Everyone Lied to Me*

*In the silence when one species is able to interact with another species, there is communion beyond our own individual intelligence. The truth is in the silence beyond our thoughts and conditioning. In no way would our collective innocence ever agree to deliberately harm a sentient soul.*

*April 12, 2017*

Day after day, I spent all my waking hours with the herd. My vision changed. I began seeing them entirely differently. I would pack a sack of raw fruit, veggies, nuts, and water and hang out with the herd from the moment I woke up to just before sundown. With a blanket strapped to my body, I trudged the acreage with the cows.

When they mooed, I mooed. When they lay down, I lay down. When they grazed, so did I—on my fruit, veggies, and nuts. I even got on all fours and nibbled at the grass. After all, humans eat cow flesh and never stop to think for one minute that cows eat grass. Their nourishment, protein, and sustenance come from grass seeds that grow in the dirt. I cringe when people say, "But where do you get your protein?"

I would munch on my food, and uncontrollable tears would fall down my cheeks as I remembered that I used to eat their bodies without a second thought. I loved to eat their ribs, their flank, and their rump. I loved brisket and stew flesh carved off their upper leg.

Pot roast, smothered steak, and ground beef are all come from the flesh of the "chuck." Another favorite of mine was chicken-fried steak carved off their shank. My favorite "cut," filet mignon, is carved from the tenderloin. It's cut from the narrow front part of their body, near the short loin.

*What changed?* In the past, I could talk about these body parts with no emotion. I was so brainwashed. But now I felt immense pain.

*Was I going crazy?*

I'm sure I looked crazy, but it didn't stop me.

I was one of them. Yes, I had a different body, but my body and their bodies felt the same emotions.

*Their bodies belonged to them, not to us.*

I observed the way they cared for each other, the way they moved harmoniously together, the incredible senses they had, much more heightened than my own. Only in the stillness and silence could I perceive this.

I pictured myself sectioned off and sold by the pound. Bodies are bodies. Flesh is flesh. We all have beating hearts, reproductive organs, and a central nervous system. All creatures feel joy, contentment, pain, suffering, and grief.

I began to practice the art of observation and silence while with the herd. I watched them one by one. I noticed their distinct personalities, the shapes of their head, eyes, ears, noses, etcetera. I noted unique markings and sounds, and their names began to emerge. I began to see them as *who*, not *what*, they were.

When we see them, *really* see them, we can't eat them. We can't put a price on them.

We bred cows to make money. That was our business. We sent the babies to sale barns when they were six to seven months old, *over* and *over* again. The momma cows were never allowed the dignity of living out their lives with their children. We betrayed the mommas and their babies time after time. We scarcely noticed their grief. Their anguish was never validated. We just used them as commodities. We considered ourselves "good stewards" and family cattle ranchers. We never doubted that our jobs were noble. But I learned that my loyalty was misplaced. Instead of being loyal to my innate compassion, I had been conditioned to accept animal agriculture as law.

Like it or not, if you eat animals, it isn't because you were born to be a flesh eater. We're conditioned by "animal ag," and it runs deep in families, especially in 4-H, a US-based network of youth organizations, FFA (Future Farmers of

America), the church, our schools, and our governments. And y'all, nobody does it better than Texas.

We are programmed to believe that it is OK for us to "own" animals. If we own them, we can decide which ones we eat and which ones are pets. God created animals to experience their own lives. The word "anima" means "soul." Contrary to my Christian upbringing, animals *do* have souls. I know it because I have felt their souls intertwined with my own.

I had to find a way to make Tommy and everyone else in Texas see what I saw.

Observing their behavior day in and day out sharpened my awareness of their individuality. As my perception of them changed, I began to focus on their family units and the community they shared. The momma cows always had babies or were pregnant because, as a cow/calf operation, that's what we did on our land.

The first time I witnessed Tippy act as the official herd babysitter, I was dumbfounded. One by one, Tippy would relieve the momma cows so that they could go and take care of themselves. Tippy would not leave their babies' side until their respective mommas returned from their grazing and water break. Then, Tippy would walk over to the next momma to relieve her until each one was taken care of. Witnessing this profound relationship changed me on the spot. How had I not seen that before?

I remember my childhood babysitter, Carol. She used to melt multicolored Lifesaver candies and give them to us as "medicine." I'll never forget her. My momma could leave *our bodies* in her care, go to work or wherever, and come back knowing that her kids were gonna be OK.

Imagine to Momma's horror if Carol had sold us kids off, or worse—mutilated us. What a nightmare.

That was not the case with the babies in our care as cattle ranchers. We never thought twice about what happened to them when they left us. We got our paycheck and went on about our "business." I can't imagine being betrayed time and time again by those I trusted.

When I realized, in the summer of 1991, that I couldn't have babies, I was devastated. The thought of never feeling a baby growing in my womb made me feel unbearable grief and despair. My body yearned to have that sacred experience with Tommy. Instinctively, I craved the experience of nurturing a child at my breast. And I imagined: *What if I was that mother with the same instincts? Then finally, I had a child, and that child that I yearned for was ripped from my side, or killed in front of me.*

Most don't notice the yearning and cries of the momma cows. I remember the way I felt when I realized I would never be able to conceive. The deep, guttural pain that came through my body was unrecognizable. I had never felt such a loss.

I began to identify with the loss that the momma cows experience. *Would my family turn their hearts, and souls away from my emotional distress if my baby was ripped from my side? Would they pretend that my feelings didn't matter?*

That's what we did to those momma cows over and over again.

The truth of who they were as grieving mommas was always right in front of me, but all I knew back then was that we were cattle ranchers and "feeding the world." Most traditional ranchers don't notice their deep yearning and cries, but they played like a chorus in my mind. This was not stewardship.

As I watched them graze, I'd rack my brain and wonder how I could be a good steward—a steward of life and not of death.

*What am I going to do now?*

I began reading Dr. Will Tuttle's book, *The World Peace Diet*[1], where I learned that our stock market was built on the backs of animals—*you know, liveSTOCK.* Capitalism was based on per capita "per head," as in per animal head.

That's when it hit me like a freight train: *Our entire capitalistic society is fundamentally built on exploiting animals.* It's not just part of the system; it's the foundation. It's what made capitalism and the brutality of animals possible.

Animals are enslaved, traded, and bred for profit on a massive scale.

Tuttle writes, "Historically, the original meaning of *war* in many early cultures, especially Indo-European, was literally 'fighting for cattle.'"

War was born from the greed for cows.

In Sanskrit, the word for animal is *paśu*, and the word *lobha* refers to greed or covetous desire. *Paśulobha* expresses a greed for animals.

*Paśulobha* is like a poison root that winds itself around and binds our hearts and chokes our deeper knowing. It threads through our lives, our families, our cultures, our traditions—normalizing violence.

These are chillingly accurate words when you're talking about the historical and modern mindset of commodifying animals. Not only does it treat animals as commodities, but that normalized violence is now treating humans and our planet as commodities. This is what we are up against.

I believe greed for animals is the seed of violence and all suffering. Domination is inevitable.

Dominion over animals or other people, for that matter, should not mean torture, abuse, and killing. I believe God's dominion is love, just as a king's dominion is stewardship. We considered ourselves stewards of these animals. We truly believed we cared for them well, but we also saw them as resources, not beings. They padded our income and filled our bellies. They died not so we could live, but so we could live more comfortably. What kind of stewardship was that? God implores us to care for His creation, not sell it, kill it, or consume it. Standing among the herd, learning from them, I saw their true glory and His. Job 12:7–10 says.

> But ask the beasts, and they will teach you; the birds of the heavens, and they will tell you; or the bushes of the earth, and they will teach you; and the fish of the sea will declare to you. Who among all these does not know that the hand of the Lord has done this? In his hand is the life of every living thing and the breath of all mankind.

Humanity's dominion should reflect God's love for His creation.

How the cows in our herd today have survived is beyond me. Agape, our twenty-six-year-old blind cow, still bears the memories and heartache of all the babies we stole from her. She was the guardian of the herd. She would charge us in a heartbeat if we got too close to her or her babies. Still, she and others in our herd were broken time and time again as we stole what was not ours to take so we could be "good cattle ranchers." As I began to see the world from their point of view, I began to see us, the humans, as their demons.

Yet here they all were, letting me into their world. My very presence emitted a deep longing for their forgiveness. I would take long walks with them into the woods. They changed me. I was undoing my programming day by day, week by week, month by month. They knew I had changed. Their grace for me, gave me grace for myself.

I felt a deep, steadying resolve and the emergence of a new role. I would defend the animals we used to breed and sell, and I would show others what the cows had shown me. The conflicts between me and Tommy escalated, but my new mission felt like a gift from God. There was no way around it. I saw cows as individuals like me. Tommy saw them as his commodities. We were at war. I knew by now that war was built on the greed of cows, and I wasn't about to surrender.

My war with Tommy was built from that same ancient fire that led men into battle to own cattle. But my fight was to free them, not to own them.

# 14

# *The Mad Cowgirl Meets the Mad Cowboy*

*My husband Tommy is a man of high integrity and respect. He believes that everything he does is to honor the land, the animals, and his ancestors. He's always been convinced that he was a humane rancher. Gradually, moment by moment, as I stay the course, his eyes and heart are opening. One thing I've learned most of all is that I have to be as compassionate toward my husband, as I am toward the cows.*

*December 21, 2014*

I spent the next several weeks afraid that Tommy would go behind my back when I wasn't looking and take all the cows to slaughter. He wasn't about to surrender his herd to me, and I'd be damned if I was gonna let him send the cows off without a showdown. I would sleep with one eye open if I had to.

Well, that's just about what it came to. We were saying things to each other that were so hateful and damaging. Words that I never would have forgiven Tommy for had I not known that my transition to veganism had shattered his entire belief system.

We were living in two separate worlds yet in the same home, on the same land, and with the same cows that were, in his mind, his business. In my mind, they were my family. By God, I was ready to do anything to keep him from killing those cows. I would've taken a bullet in the street on Highway 35 if he had crossed me!

I kept praying for wisdom, and then I checked Facebook.

I joined a group there called the Global Vegan Registry, where I started privately messaging my first vegan friend, Jeanne Westphal, from Crescent City, California. She inspired me to write about our dilemma and start a secret diary on Facebook called *The Vegan Journal of a Cattle Rancher's Wife*. I amassed a following faster than I ever could have ever imagined.

Our story was outrageous, and it reminded my new vegan friends about an icon of former-cattle-ranching named Howard Lyman. I had never heard of him, but I was intrigued. The more I learned, the more determined I became to meet him.

Mr. Lyman was a fourth-generation cattle rancher raised on a farm that produced dairy and meat commodities. He graduated from Montana State University in 1961 with a BS in general agriculture. Mr. Lyman was actively engaged in animal and grain production for two decades. His business included dairy, pork, registered Hereford beef, chicken, range cattle, feedlot beef production, veal, grain, silage, and hay production.

As fate would have it, Mr. Lyman was diagnosed with a tumor in his spine in 1979. That tumor led him to follow his heart, mind, and soul, eventually leading him to veganism and selling his animal agriculture business. His investigations in 1989 led him to believe that the roots of many health concerns around eating meat were due to mad cow disease.

Mad cow disease slowly destroys the cattle's brain and spinal cord and is fatal. The technical terminology for mad cow disease is bovine spongiform encephalopathy (BSE). Cows get this disease by eating feed contaminated with the body parts of other cows infected with BSE.

In 1996, Mr. Lyman spoke out about mad cow on national TV. He was even on the *Oprah Winfrey Show*. His remarks about BSE, such as "mad cow disease would make AIDS look like the common cold," exposed animal agriculture and led Oprah to publicly renounce hamburgers. This pissed off the National Cattlemen's Beef Association so much that they sued both Mr. Lyman and Oprah. Both were found not guilty in 1998, and beef was in the news in a terrible light for the first time ever.

Mr. Lyman was launched into the limelight as an animal rights activist. He was featured in many of the documentaries that Jeanne recommended I watch. I even read his book *The Mad Cowboy*.

By December 2014, I was desperate to talk to him. I knew that it was only a matter of time before fate would intervene and our paths would cross. He felt like the only person in the whole wide world who could understand where I was coming from. Certainly, he would support my plan, and I was determined to win his favor so that he could help me influence Tommy to renounce cattle ranching, see my point of view, and go vegan.

It took several failed calls and emails before he finally picked up the phone on Christmas Eve, 2014. Some things remain in your brain forever. I was frantic to talk to him. Having no one to talk to about all of this had been terrifying and isolating. I needed guidance. I know I had people like Jeanne and my Facebook group followers, but no one understood what it felt like to be in the cattle ranching business and go through a vegan transition. I felt like I was losing my mind. I was all bottled-up anger and rage. I wanted to lash out at Tommy whenever he opened his mouth.

Until I talked to Mr. Lyman, I told the cows about my heartbreak and betrayal. I spent hours with the herd, crying and screaming, and they would just chew their cud, flex their ears and brow, and look at me as if they understood. I would lay flat on my back with my arms and legs wide in the middle of the pasture with the cows all around me. It was as if they all knew what was about to happen next.

I would pack my lunch, take a thermos, a blanket, and my guitar, and off I would go to reflect and *be* with my cow family. The more I knew them, the more I knew I had to reach Mr. Lyman. There was no way in hell that I could ever let these animals go to the sale barn.

During those long hours in the pasture, when I'd lie in the grass with my arms outstretched like a starfish, soaking up all the vibes of Mother Earth and surrounded by my cow family, I started thinking about how I was conceived in violence.

I thought about my momma—and what she told me happened when she was just sixteen. A child. Her own innocence was stolen by a man twice her age. A so-called family friend. His wife, Barbara, had taken her own life, and while he was still grieving, he took my momma to the cemetery where Barbara was buried—and raped her there.

*That man would become my father.*

It was betrayal in its rawest form. A violation of sacred trust. And here I was, decades later, reliving that grief—but now it was through the eyes of the cows. They looked at me like I was their protector, their safe place. But we were raising them for slaughter. But no more.

I told them that day that I would do whatever I had to in order to end the cycle of betrayal.

By then, I was a brand new vegan. The veil had been lifted, and I was wide awake in a world I didn't know how to live in yet. I couldn't unsee what I saw. And I sure as hell couldn't pretend I didn't feel it. So I told the cows everything—about my broken trust with Tommy, about the storms raging inside of me, and about my momma. I cried with those cows. And they just stood there, calm and knowing, chewing their cud like they were holding space for me or something. Like they understood.

The pasture became my vision board. It was there that I started visualizing the cows safe in a sanctuary.

*Do I dare dream that these cows could be safe, right here? Could this be sacred ground?*

I'd beg God to show me how to save the herd.

And I made a promise out there in the dirt among the cow patties—they would not go to the sale barn! *Over my dead body.* Not ever.

Vegan for three months, and sober for just a little over a year, I began to see that I would have to bust through this cycle of violence to be true to myself.

*If I am going to stay sober, I have to break this curse. If I go back to the way it's always been... Renée gets drunk.*

In AA, we talk about doing "the next right thing," so I had no doubt in my mind that staying sober and saving the cows was *the next right thing.*

I didn't know how, but I was going to keep suiting up and showing up (my sponsor would add shut up and grow up). So, this was me growing up.

## A Pivotal Phone Call

Mr. Lyman finally answered the phone on Christmas Eve as I stood over the stove cooking my first Christmas side dishes without milk, eggs, cheese, or animal flesh. Tommy was in the living room, so I sped by to talk privately to Mr. Lyman.

"Watch the stove," I yelled as I ran to the bedroom and slammed the door behind me.

With a slow, deliberate drawl, Mr. Lyman said, "You must be Renée."

"How did you know?" I exclaimed.

"Well, I recognize the number since you've called me a half dozen times or more. What can I do for you?"

I immediately launched into a dramatic explanation of my plight. Every detail poured out of me in a frenzy as Mr. Lyman calmly listened to my rant. The entirety of my conversation was about telling him how horrible Tommy was and how I felt all alone. I gave him every detail of my plan. I was going to save the cows from slaughter and start a sanctuary. I had it all figured out, but I needed his advice on how to talk some sense into Tommy so he would listen and understand me.

He listened to me for about five minutes.

"Are you through?" he asked

"Yes, sir."

Calmly, he said, "Don't you think you ought to have the same compassion for Tommy as you have for those cows?"

You could've blown me over with a feather.

I was shocked that he would take up for my husband, who was so sick of the situation that he wanted to send all the cows to the sale barn, get out of the business and get a divorce.

"But Mr. Lyman, Tommy is a murderer! I can't possibly be nice to him. He needs to wake up!"

He laughed kindly, not at me.

"My dear, your husband is a good man, and it sounds like you've pretty much destroyed his world. I recommend taking a minute, being thankful for him, and trying to see things from his point of view. Slow down, listen, and just be kind to him."

He added, "If you want to start a sanctuary, I advise you to go and visit about six of them before you make that decision because it's a difficult life and one that you shouldn't make hastily."

"I can't! If I leave, Tommy will sell the cows, and I could never live with myself if these cows go to slaughter. I see them now, every one of them, as individuals. There's no way I can leave."

"Well," he said, "It looks like you've got some decisions to make. The first recommendation is to slow down, listen, and be kind to Tommy. You might also stop calling him a murderer."

It was true that I'd been, well, *rowdy* about things. Mr. Lyman had a point. If it was all about compassion, I ought to try to find some for Tommy.

Talking to Mr. Lyman eased my heart. It helped me rethink Tommy as a cattle rancher with a moral and traditional dilemma instead of a murderer. Mr. Lyman became my soft place to land with all my anger, fears, insecurities, and questions. His soft-spoken but direct approach made me listen. We've stayed in touch over the years. I will forever be in debt to his kindness as my first vegan cattle rancher mentor.

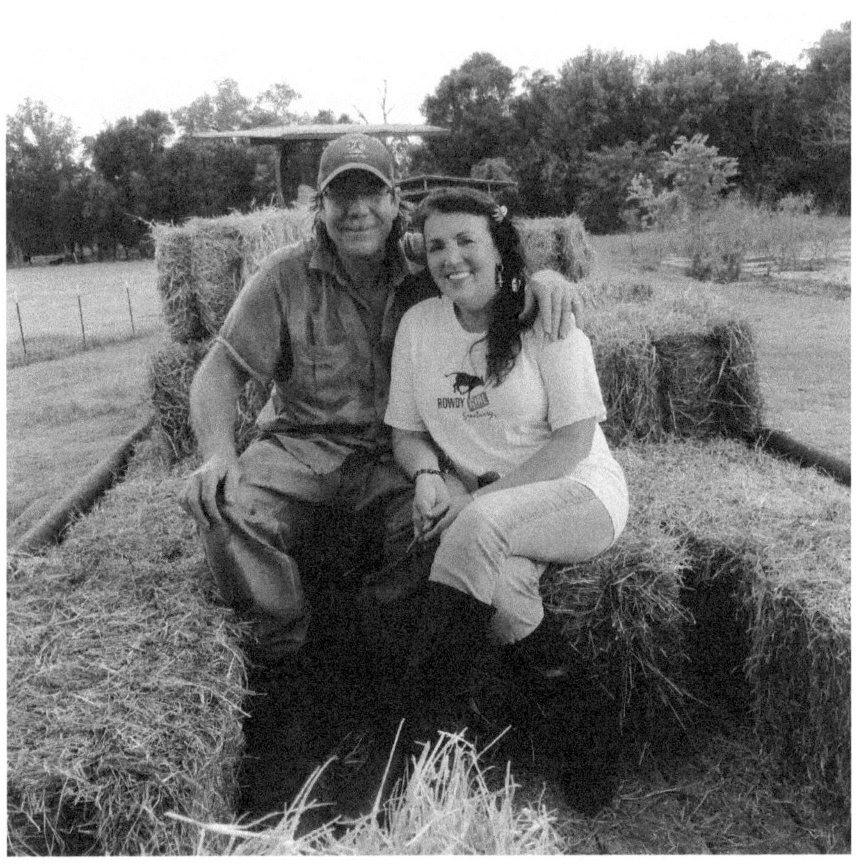


**Figure 6 Early Angleton.** *Hay bales, hard work, and a smile that masked the storms coming. We didn't yet know how much would unravel or how much we would transform.*

# 15

# *The Showdown*

*Tommy and I spend every day making the world a better place for farm animals. I am so blessed to have him as my partner in life! As October approaches I'm reminded about what it was like ten years ago. I was going crazy on a cattle ranch and Tommy was trying to figure out how to hold it all together. Now, here we are—both vegan—defying all odds!*

*September 22, 2024*

Juxtapose my Texas family upbringing and my husband's family traditions, fraught with the culture of normalized violence, and you can see how I was hanging by a thread on the edge of a cliff.

*Do I jump into the world of veganism, which I'm confident is the original intent of creation?*

*Or do I turn my back on the truth and run back into the darkness that consumed my innocence?*

I chose to jump, and I landed in the light of veganism. A new dawn had awakened upon my consciousness, and with that intense light bouncing off my aura came others seeking the light that enveloped the darkness of my soul. When the Rowdy Girl story started making its way around the globe, cattle ranchers, their families, and friends were enthralled with our conversion. We had crossed over and managed the unthinkable. We had escaped the stronghold of animal agriculture and were out on a limb of unimaginable uncertainty.

I spent the next several weeks afraid that Tommy would go behind my back when I wasn't looking and take all the cows to slaughter. He wasn't about to surrender his herd to me, and I'd be damned if I was gonna let him send the cows to slaughter without a showdown. But I kept Mr. Lyman's words close to my heart.

Tommy and I were saying things to each other that were hateful. Words that I swear I would've never forgiven Tommy for had I not known he was hanging on to every shred of the belief system he grew up in.

Humans will fight ferociously to keep their animal-eating traditional beliefs intact because they define us. Without our familial foundation of eating animals, who are we? Ask any vegan who tries to have dinner with their family after they've "crossed over," and invariably, every one of them will say something like:

*My family is so mad at me.*
*They think I've betrayed them or joined a cult.*
*They think I'm judging them.*

Tommy still had that cherished elk head hung on the wall near the apex of our high ceiling. As I said before, many a day, I visualized hanging my husband from the horns of that elk. At the time, he thought it was a cherished "family heirloom" that he should pass down to generations. After I went vegan, the thought of that elk being a "family heirloom" sickened me. I didn't want to hurt Tommy, but I did want him to evaporate, *to just go away*. But he wouldn't.

He was not about to leave his land, possessions, and cattle to me. I wasn't about to leave him because if I did, he would've sent every single cow to the slaughterhouse. We succumbed to unrelenting pressure as things got worse and worse.

I was coming up with a plan to buy Tommy's cows, take over the ranch, and transform it into a farm animal sanctuary. I had no idea how this was going to happen, but I knew it would. It was like when I got my first band together—*Renée King and Wildcard*. I didn't know how I was going to do it. I just knew, by God, I was going to do whatever it took to get it done! One day at a time, one step at a time, one follower at a time, one donation at a time—until the day that I could confront my husband and give him an ultimatum. Either he was going to let me buy his cows, or I was going to make his life a living hell.

But I needed other people's ideas and insights to help see that it was really possible. This was all new territory for me, and there was no way I could get through it on my own.

That's when I found the Global Vegan Registry on Facebook, where I met my first vegan friend, Jeanne Westphal, it was like I had found my tribe. I met people who had been ethical vegans for years. They understood my grief. I could cry my eyes out to them, and they would listen. These were some hard-core ethical vegans—the kind of vegans your momma and daddy write home about. Blood in the street types. And they were enthralled with my story.

They would become glued to the page of my brain and heart. Their accumulative beliefs in veganism fueled my activism.

I'd become so close to Jeanne. She would take my calls all through the night. She became my lifeline, and encouraged me to take my journey public.

"You start writing about this and there are people out there who will rush to help you! People are waiting right now to help you!" Jeanne told me.

Bright red hair and a million-dollar smile—and an attitude to boot—Jeanne inspired me and pushed me to go the distance. I started a secret diary and called it *Vegan Journal of a Cattle Rancher's Wife.*

Tommy was clueless.

At the time, he wasn't on Facebook so it was an easy secret to keep. Still though, I kept my conversations with Jeanne private, and my growing Global online community a secret. Not only did I need to keep it a secret from my cattle ranching husband, but I also needed to keep it from the entire Brazoria County cattle rancher community.

People around the world knew what was going on before my next-door neighbors!

As my online community grew, so did my confidence.

I struck up friendships with an American filmmaker named Kip Andersen and a vegan attorney named Robert, who helped me craft the narrative that would become my plea to the world, "Help Me Buy My Husband's Cows to Save Them from Slaughter." With their support and the rallying cries of my readers, a little campaign became a movement.

Between Kip, Robert, and Jeanne, I was ready to challenge my husband and make him an offer he couldn't refuse.

Now, mind you, I had played out this scenario time and time again with my three new vegan friends. No rancher's wife in her right mind would ever challenge a cattle rancher husband and live to talk about it, especially in Texas.

However, I was so distraught over the thought of the cows going to slaughter that I was ready to do just that. I didn't think I could live with myself if I didn't.

Only two months after going vegan, I published my plea and confronted Tommy in the pasture.

*Would I break and have a relapse into alcoholism, or worse?*

My last relapse was so bad that the very thought of it forced me into a passionate stance against my husband.

All I could hear was, *To thine own self be true.*

How could I be true to my vegan self if I let those cows die? I couldn't. So the war was on!

With every nerve firing and all the confidence I could muster, I began the conversation that would be our first step toward salvation—for both the cows and me.

On *that* day, Tommy and I were arguing loudly in the front pasture with the red trailer ready to take the cows to slaughter.

"Stay out of my god-damned business, Renée," he shouted, throwing his cap onto the ground.

"This is no longer a business," I shouted back. "These cows are my family, and if you take them up the road one more time to the sale barn, I swear to you I will follow you and buy every single one back and bring them back home using your credit card. Furthermore, if you get in my way, I will make you the most embarrassed man in Brazoria County. I'll become the kind of vegan who waves a flag and shouts into a megaphone. I'll go to jail if I have to. You will not take those cows to the sale barn!"

There was a long period of silence. My heart was beating out of my chest, and I prayed with every breath, "Thy will be done."

Finally, Tommy broke the silence and said, "What are you gonna do with my cows?"

"Well," I replied, "I'm gonna start a sanctuary. A nonprofit that saves animals from going to slaughter."

"You've lost your mind," he laughed.

"Yeah, I have and thank God! I've got a renewed mind," I told him, "The mind I lost was the one that believed eating animals was normal. My new mind is a clean slate, and I see clearly that cows are not meant to be eaten by humans. They are meant to be protected and loved."

Tommy shook his head and grinned. It was good to see him grinning

"A sanctuary for cows in Texas? There ain't no way you can do something like that."

"Well, why not?" I asked, "If there ain't one, then that means there needs to be, and we will be the first."

I got up my nerve and pounced.

"How about I make a deal with you?" I continued, "If you're gonna sell all the cows anyway, why don't you sell 'em to me?"

"Sell 'em to *you*?" he gasped. "You've got to be kidding me! How are you gonna buy my cows?"

It was then that I 'fessed up and told him all about my secret diary on Facebook. I told him all about the thousands of followers I had amassed after a few days and that I was ready to launch a fundraiser if he would just give me permission to buy his cows.

I'll never forget the look on his face when I told him this story. He put his hand on his head, slowly shaking it, mouth wide open—totally dumbfounded. Then he lost it. But he wasn't angry, he thought it was hilarious.

"Those words don't even go together… buy… my… cows?" He paused and thought: *All this time, Renée had been behind my back scheming to buy my cows*?

It was preposterous. That really got him laughing hysterically.

Tommy rarely laughs out loud, but this gave him a big ol' belly laugh, and he couldn't stop. He thought it was the funniest thing he had ever heard.

Finally, he regained his composure and said sarcastically, "You want to buy my cows? OK, I could get $35,000–40,000 for 'em at the sale barn because several of them are pregnant and have babies that can be sold as a cow/calf pair."

"Well, how much will you sell 'em to your wife for," I asked, serious as a heart attack. I could tell by the look in his eyes that Tommy no more believed I would pull off buying his cows than I could put a man on the moon.

He decided to go with it. "I'll sell 'em to you for $30,000," he said, playing along.

"Will you let me lease the land for $1 a year?"

"Sure," he kidded.

"How about for two years?" I bargained.

"You got a deal," he said, and shook my hand.

The rest as they say… *is herstory.*

Tears flooded my eyes. I'd never been more relieved in my life. I gave Tommy a big hug. He didn't hug me back, but I knew he would one day. We had a deal, and Tommy Sonnen isn't the type of man who ever backs down on his word.

# 16

# *The Sacred Bond of Violence*

*I am finding my strength, or I should say that it has found me. Some days I feel inadequate to be birthing this mission and then I remember that Rowdy Girl Sanctuary is not about me; it is coming through me. I've had no children of my own, but I know that children come through the birth canal they do not belong to the Mother—the Mother is to be the caregiver, the nurturer, the light and persistent strength that gracefully yields so that the infant can come through.*

*April 15, 2015*

We shook on it. I was going to buy Tommy's cows. He wouldn't dare go back on his word, but that didn't stop him from dealing a last ditch emotional bargaining chip.

"Renée, if we do this, you can never have that baby you want," Tommy said. "If you forget about this crazy notion of turning our ranch into a sanctuary, you can go ahead and start the paperwork for getting a baby for us to raise as our own."

It felt like emotional blackmail at the eleventh hour. It was designed to stop me in my tracks.

It gutted me that he would hang the one thing I wanted more than anything in the world over my head—a baby *with him*. But when faced with the thought of having a baby at the cost of killing the cows, I knew I was doing the right thing. I had grown to love Rowdy Girl and all the cows. They had become my family. He didn't know it yet, but one day, they'd be his family too.

He violated a bond that I wanted to have with him. I wanted it with him. My soul was violated.

Despite the fact that I ached to have a child with him, I pressed on to save the cows.

I launched the campaign in January of 2015, and money started rolling in. It wasn't easy, but I wasn't alone. Community was critical; it *is* critical in any kind of movement. Every single dollar donated and word of encouragement lifted my heart. I wasn't crazy, there were people all over the world who wanted to see this happen.

Tommy and I still argued daily. I still yelled at him when he talked about selling the cows and he still tried everything to get me to reconsider. Tommy was very apprehensive and not yet a vegan. His whole life had been founded on principles that shored up "animal ag" and hunting. He was embarrassed and had a lot of resentment toward me for wrecking his perfect retirement portfolio. The movement was bigger than his pissed off cow-loving wife. It wasn't just me changing; people all over the world were. He would never say it, but I'm sure it scared the living hell outta him.

My husband had built a comfortable ranching life at the tail end of his career at Dow Chemical. It was a natural choice—the career of his forefathers. He wanted to finally work outdoors, have a career that didn't box him in, and be the master of his own schedule. And now he was watching it all unravel.

Tommy's whole life had been founded on principles that shored up "animal ag" and hunting. He had a lot of resentment toward me for wrecking his perfect retirement portfolio. He begrudgingly trudged forward day by day into the holiday season—a season of great relief for me and one of bittersweet "days gone by" for my husband.

This is why he was so desperate to cling to this way of life, why he had the audacity to throw the promise of a child in my face if I would forget my crazy dream of having a sanctuary for cows. The only reason he resorted to such extreme manipulation was because of the sacred bond that cattle ranchers have with each other—the bond of allowing violence toward animals as acceptable and normal. He was willing to manipulate me to go against my newfound vegan ethics so he could prop up tradition.

## What Is That Bond?

We live in an illusion. Society is entrenched in false beliefs that carry us through our entire existence. We build family structures on ideals cemented through the annals of time. Take a quick look at family photo albums, and you can easily see the patterns of animal cruelty rooting and taking shape in the lives of innocent children, poised in the guise of family tradition.

When Tommy and I married the first time, we spent a lot of time in West Texas. Tommy had property in Junction, and he used to hunt *a lot*. Let's just say I had a hallway in our house that we nicknamed "the horny hall."

All his friends were hunters. All they ever talked about was how many points were on the racks of the deer they hunted, ate, and showcased. I remember listening to tales of "buck fever" and how excited and amped up the men would get as they relished the memories of their kills. These acts of blatant violence were the bonding agents of their manhood and friendship.

Of course, I didn't see it that way at the time. I was enthralled. As one of the women on the outside, I felt privileged to be allowed into their private world of manly pursuits. Early in the morning, before the sun came up, the guys would all gather around the campfire, their breath steamy from the freezing temperatures. Sipping their fireside coffee in a silent ceremony, they quietly assembled for their quest. Equipped with camo, combat boots, guns, and rugged gear, they prepared to kill.

It was a silent meditation and ritual bound in ancient memories of the past. It played out before me like a preordained script. Their fathers, grandfathers, and great-grandfathers had passed down this sacred ceremony that prepared the men for the hunt, roused their thirst for blood to come in the dawning hours.

I recalled the stacks of photo albums filled with the smiling faces of grown men, grasping the antlers of warm bodies. I never wondered then what was to become of the families left behind. I do now.

The young boys with the men anxiously awaited their rite of passage. The photos of six- to seven-year-old boys emulating their fathers, uncles, and other role models still haunt me. Now that I'm vegan, I can't imagine how loving families could adopt such a violent tradition.

How did we come to believe that killing innocent animals in their homes was sacred? The most haunting photos were those of young boys with faces painted with the blood of their first kill. The blood-smeared, proud smile of a child surrounded by his peers was a cherished memory for them. That photo sealed the deal. Their first kill was a spiritual consecration. They were now officially ordained a "man."

*How did we ever twist and turn the love of God's creation into this?*

This photo is one of the first in a painful thread. Images that quietly reveal how violence becomes normalized and is even revered within the family unit.

These young men would grow up to be cattle ranchers, game wardens, and FFA dads. The traditions of sacred violence have shaped the ranching culture of the modern day.

The day I turned on Tommy and went vegan, I slapped him and his family square in the spiritual face of a tradition that generations upheld. Going vegan on your cattle rancher husband was a "sin," which, according to the Oxford English dictionary, is "an immoral act considered to be a transgression against divine law." That is precisely how Tommy, his family, and my mother must've seen my transgression.

I remember people shaming me, "Renée, how could you do that to your husband? You ought to be ashamed of yourself!" Me? Ashamed of myself? My new vegan spiritual experience was fresh and innocent. Every assault against the emerging "unadulterated truth" consumed my consciousness. I felt it as a searing hot iron upon my sensitive soul. How could they think that not killing animals was an act of insubordination? They all agreed that my decision to align with the gentlest part of my soul was a crime and a sin against my husband.

While with Tommy and his hunting brethren, I remembered climbing up into the tree where a freshly killed deer was hanging. I turned this gruesome act of violence into an anatomy and physiology lesson while they did what hunters call "field dressing." From a bird's eye view, I watched with great interest every single move the hunter's blade made while they pulled off the deer's hide with razor precision and opened her bowels from the anus to her chest to allow her guts to pour out onto the ground.

The first step in cooling the flesh was removing the deer's internal organs. When the bowels and blood fell to the ground, the smell and warmth of her innards consumed me. I still remember the smell mixed with the grass that was her last meal. As part of my own cognitive dissonance, I had to experience the act of turning this beautiful wild deer, a mother with her young alone in the wilderness, into food for people who had other options.

Never once did I consider that this mother's fawn was peering from behind a tree, watching while her only chance for survival was being bagged and tagged for deer sausage.

*How could I have become so seduced by evil that killing became normalized in my thoughts, words, and deeds?*

Money, greed, profit, control, and spiritual warfare—*that's how.*

Consider for a moment what the Bible really means when it speaks about the "lust of the flesh." Lust can take any form, such as lust for sexuality, money, or power. It can take on such mundane forms as the lust for food, distinct from the "need" for food, or redolence when someone lusts for a particular smell that brings back memories.

We find in 1 John 2:16, "For everything in the world—the lust of the flesh, the lust of the eyes, and the pride of life—comes not from the Father but from the world."

Ponder for a moment that the enemy that keeps us bound in the darkness of normalized violence does so by seducing the masses with physical gratification. We become preoccupied with it, whether it's sex, drugs, alcohol, or whether we crave bodies of flesh. Throughout the Bible, man was tempted by evil.

What makes any of us think now that the same temptations are not rampant among us? Our Creator never condoned animal agriculture. As God's children, He created us to be good stewards over His Earth and His animals. He charged us to have dominion over them, not to dominate the Earth and the animals, and to profit off them or violate their rights as fellow creatures.

Animal agriculture is rooted in evil. In my experience, the very personal awakening I had living on a Texas cattle ranch was akin to the moment I was "born again" when I first encountered a spiritual experience with Jesus. Only dying to "the flesh" now had a new meaning for me. I truly did die to "the flesh"—the flesh of animals as food. There was nothing symbolic about it.

My hope for you reading this book is that you, too, will have your own spiritual awakening and will no longer need to eat dead bodies to feel alive. The very idea that the death of animals equals life in our bodies is perverted. I was brought up to believe that the final sacrifice was Jesus. His death on the cross should mean that no animal would ever have to die again for humans to crave their burnt flesh.

The sacred idol of the "golden calf" was now abolished once and for all. I believe that the true mystery of the "golden calf," back in the days of Moses, was twofold. At that time, man lusted after wealth and burnt offerings. The lust for gold and meat was their symbolic idol. To this day, it is still considered sacred. The roots of our violent twentieth-century culture run deep.

I leave you with this nursery rhyme that resonates wherever I go for the animals.

*This little light of mine, I'm gonna let it shine. This little light of mine, I'm gonna let it shine. This little light of mine, I'm gonna let it shine, let it shine, let it shine, let it shine.*

# 17

# *Tinseltown in Angleton*

*Animal agriculture should have NEVER become an industrialized or mechanized killing machine. We should have NEVER started down this path of breeding, commodifying and killing animals for profit, and to dominate the world. But we have.*

*May 12, 2023*

Around late February 2015, just when we thought everything was going perfectly, a group of filmmakers approached us about telling our story in a well-funded documentary. We were still in the fundraising stages and the producers' promises appealed to my desperate need to raise money to save the cows.

We were close to reaching our goal, but you need every push you can get when you're a cattle rancher's wife trying to buy your husband's cows. We were an anomaly.

Thankfully, Tommy and I were in this sweet spot where he had finally come to terms with the fact that his cattle ranch was close to becoming a vegan farm sanctuary. He wasn't yet vegan, but he was convinced that the vegan community was on our side as the funds poured in.

The filmmakers were smart and flashy, and they seemed as passionate about the sanctuary as we were. They sold the concept of the film to us by saying they loved our story, their executive producers would spare no expense to give Tommy and me what we needed to make the farm successful. They promised new barns, equipment, fencing, whatever we could dream of. We just had to sell them our beautiful story of a cattle ranch transitioning to a vegan farm.

"You'll have to sign a nondisclosure agreement," they said. "It will bind you for five years from telling anybody the names of the executive producers."

Since this is *my* diary, I'm gonna shoot it to ya straight—I've got zero interest in dragging these folks through the mud. We've thrived without the likes of them and their shady promises. But let's be honest, there's always a rotten apple in the bunch—even in the vegan movement. Some of them aren't even vegan—they just circle like vultures, ready to exploit the real ones doing the work.

In the middle of a critical time in my relationship with Tommy, this unethical film company tried to come between us. And no one is going to come between me and Tommy—except the cows!

With desperation in my bones, Tommy and I signed the NDA and moved forward with production. At the time, it felt like an answered prayer. It was a chance to take care of our cows in style, tell our story, and maybe even shake things up a bit. So, Tinseltown came on down to Angleton.

The filmmakers came to the ranch several times to film me and Tommy, both together and separately. They spent many days filming and schmoozing with us while weaving a fairytale fantasy of how all our needs would be met at the end of the day when the executive producers chose our story. They were so convincing.

They filmed a music video of me singing a song that I wrote about The Red Trailer after I went vegan. The same one that used to haunt me, the same one that used to take all those babies to the sale barn. For the shoot, I brought my guitar, my voice, and *everything* in me, and they brought all the bells and whistles—microphones, cameras, and lights like I was going to be performing on the famous stage of the Grand Ole Opry or something. I belted my song from inside the Red Trailer. It was no longer a vehicle of death; it was a symbol of hope.

They promised us that, no matter what happened, they would allow us to use the video on our website. At least they kept that promise. That's about the only damn promise they kept.

That music video is still on our Rowdy Girl Website by the way.[1] When you get a minute, check it out!

However, along with that promise came many other carrot-dangling nuances of hope that never materialized, because my husband chose *the road less traveled.*

Unbeknownst to us at the time, they were trying to pit me and Tommy against each other. They'd been manipulating us. It was all high drama and orchestration. When they were filming Tommy and me separately, they were trying to determine whether or not Tommy would be willing to become a "humane" cattle ranch instead of a sanctuary! *What the hell?*

You know the kind—-those serene, pastoral scenes you glimpse from rural highways and country roads. But behind the quiet charm lies a hidden reality: a system of violence—that sacred bond—that ultimately betrays the very bovine beings they are "humanely raising."

These filmmakers never wanted me to raise the funds to buy my husband's cows. *Never*. Meanwhile, they were filling my head with ideas of grandeur. They were positioning me to feel excited about the possibility of their executive producer helping turn our cattle ranch into a beautiful vegan sanctuary complete with everything Tommy and I could ever need.

Secretly, they were hoping that our fundraiser would fall apart. That way, they could swoop in and save the day by turning our struggling cattle ranch into another kind of cattle ranch, ultimately partnering with a company committed to killing our cows for humane meat. We were bamboozled.

After weeks of filming, we hit a huge fundraising milestone. I was inches away from owning the herd. Then, everything went silent from the filmmakers. Crickets.

I was excited we were raising the money. Hallelujah! The first beef cattle ranch in the world was about to become a vegan sanctuary! I called the filmmakers repeatedly, leaving message after message, but no one called me back.

"What happened?" I pondered. "Why won't they call me back?"

Eventually, one of the filmmakers finally called me back. I was so excited to hear from them, and tell them that we had raised the money. I put them on speaker so Tommy could hear too.

"Well," she said, "Since your fundraiser worked, the executive producers have decided to go a different route. They want to tell the story of a family cattle ranch becoming a 'humane meat' farm."

I'm not the kinda person who gets high blood pressure, but at this moment it was at an all-time high. I couldn't believe what I was hearing. Heartbreak, fury, and betrayal flooded over me all in one moment. I had expected their reaction to be congratulations and support for raising the money, but instead it was betrayal.

She continued, "Simultaneously, we've been filming another family, and the producers have chosen to go with them. Their story better fits our business model."

We had no idea about the other family. They had been stringing us along the whole time. As soon as I raised the money, they didn't want anything to do with us.

Then she said something even more shocking.

"If, however, you and Tommy want to transition to a 'humane' beef cattle ranch, the executive producers would be thrilled to tell your story, but from what I've seen on social media, y'all are happy to be a vegan sanctuary."

I was so angry. They didn't want a story that challenged the system. They wanted one that propped it up. All this time, they were rooting for our failure, expecting us to buckle. We didn't. So our story was scrapped. All that buildup, and then… nothing.

My heartbeat intensified, and I could hardly breathe. Tears rushed to my eyes, and I flushed. I was speechless, but Tommy's pre-vegan voice spoke up.

"No deal." he said, "You tell them they are unethical, and the answer is *no*!"

"I can't believe this is happening." I said shakily.

At that point, I was sobbing. All the dreams they had convinced me would come to pass faded into nothingness. The filmmaker apologetically said her goodbyes and wished us luck. That was that.

Their intention was never to tell the feel-good story of a cattle ranch going vegan. All along, they hoped to tell the story of a small, privately owned cattle ranch partnering with a corporate giant that would serve their insatiable desire to exploit cattle in animal agriculture's "humane meat" racket.

After I got off the phone, Tommy and I looked at each other in disbelief. At that moment, I knew my husband was all the way in. He wasn't quite vegan yet, but he was in. He could've gone to the dark side at that moment. We could've had all the money we could ever ask for to give our humble ranch a beautiful facelift—barns, fences, equipment, infrastructure. They knew they couldn't buy me, which was no surprise, but they could not buy Tommy either.

Later, Tommy confessed that the filmmakers took him back into the woods and filmed him for a long time, bombarding him with baited questions and ideas to make him reconsider whether he was happy converting from a small beef cattle ranch to a vegan sanctuary. They told Tommy, "We'll bring a big crew of people in here and make this farm shine."

The carrots these filmmakers dangled throughout filming led us to believe they truly wanted to showcase our transition story. Yes, they were always a little vague, but they never missed a chance to tell us how much money we'd receive *if* the executive producers picked us. What they didn't say—*what they never even hinted at*—was that the real story they were chasing was one of betrayal.

Tommy thinks there's a slush fund of money somewhere that hires people to sabotage folks like us who are making a big difference. Maybe it's Big Ag or maybe it's some other group of people afraid of systemic change. Ever since then, Tommy's been sure that animal agriculture has its tentacles all over the animal rights movement in disguise. He'll talk your ear off about it.

You can't build a movement alone, but you really have to be careful who you trust. You have to keep an eye out for promises that seem too good to be true. We've been preyed on more than a few times over the years by the likes of "would-be" vegan heroes who have no real profile. They claim to be allies, but relentlessly try to sabotage us and other animal rights organizations that are making significant headway in changing the culture of the world. We've even been written about as an organization to "watch" in multiple animal agriculture journals. You gotta have tough skin to survive in animal rights as a nonprofit. So far, we've passed the test and keep on going despite the odds.

What if Tommy had said yes? Rowdy Girl, Houdini, and all of the other bovines in our original herd would be in the butcher section of a well-known grocery store chain specializing in "humane meat." The thought of it mortifies me. I was so proud of Tommy. That's when I knew there was nothing that was going to shake Tommy's resolve. He no longer followed the money.

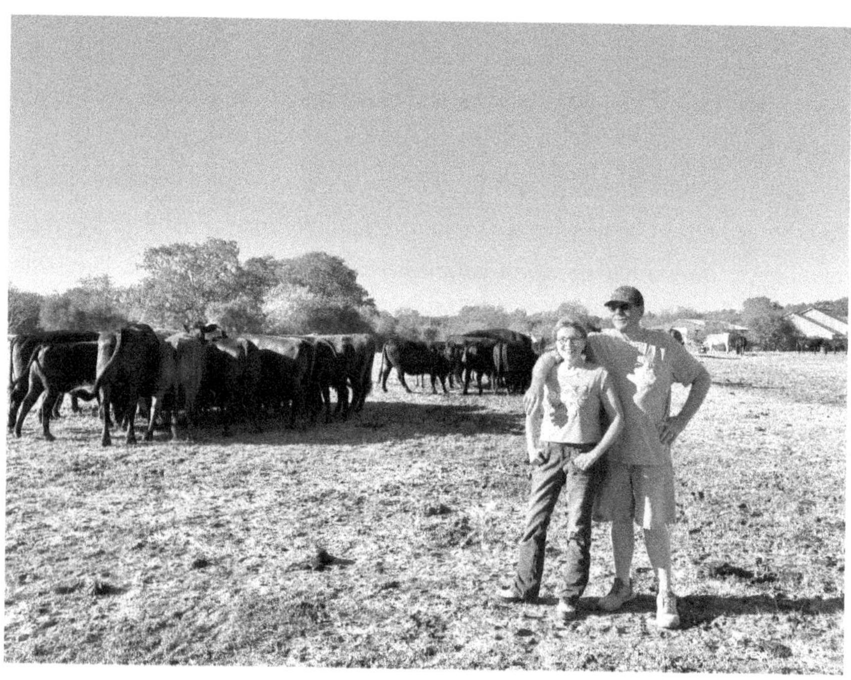

**Figure 7 Renée, Tommy, and the Herd.** *The family we never expected, and the one that pulled us from the life of cattle ranchers into the rescue story we were meant to live.*

# 18

# *From Ranch to Rescue*

*The time has come! We are now an official NONPROFIT cleared by the IRS. How exciting it is to have come all the way with you in my journal. It is right here where I began my journey on December 20, 2014. I was a distracted and scared rancher's wife gone vegan. I feared my marriage was coming apart at the seams. I was seeing the cows in our pastures through the eyes of love and compassion and was passionately doing all I could to save them from slaughter.*

*July 14, 2015*

On February 20, 2015, Rowdy Girl Sanctuary, Inc. got its official 501c3 nonprofit status. Life has been crazy since the day I went vegan in 2014. My life became a whirlwind, driven by a power greater than myself. We were positioned to be the world's first *documented* beef cattle ranch to go vegan and live to tell about it. I'm not claiming we were the first, but we *are* the first to come out, speak up, and document the journey. And that's a fact!

There were bad apples, but there were many more good ones, our tireless champions, just regular people, who donated what they could and shared our story. CBS Evening News' *Steve Hartman on the Road* came to see us, as well as other media outlets such as the *Texas Country Reporter*, *Animal Planet*, and even Southwest Airlines. Next thing I knew, Rowdy Girl Sanctuary went viral.

With that sudden attention came much love and admiration from the vegan community, and we also met with some interesting resistance—not from cattle ranchers, but from a few *unhinged crazy vegans*. In our vegan world, I learned that buying animals was a no-no, but who knew? I didn't! All I knew was that if

I didn't buy my husband's cows, they would all go to slaughter, and I was ready to put my entire life, and Tommy's, on the line to save them all.

Animal rights and farm sanctuary politics *are* a thing, but I don't play those kinds of games. We don't have time to waste playing politics when there's so much work to be done. I am here to save lives and not stroke egos. So, when the Uglies started coming after me, claiming I was using the good nature of the vegan community to create a "get rich quick scheme," I was shocked.

It showed me just how threatened some people are when you disrupt the system—*and succeed.* I broke the cardinal rule—don't buy animals from the system. It's an unspoken rule that vegans don't buy animals from the system because it reinforces the system. But all I knew was that those cows had become my family. There was no way I could have sent those cows to market. As a freshly ethical vegan, I had to buy them myself. Tommy wasn't going to give 'em to me! He had to pay taxes, balloon notes coming due, insurance payments, tractor notes, equipment bills, etcetera.

"You've got to be kidding me!" I thought.

The easier, softer way would've been for me to just let Tommy buy and sell the cows, as he'd always done, save my marriage, and travel the world after Tommy retired from Dow Chemical.

*Give me a break!*

I was becoming more like Rowdy Girl with every passing day—no longer willing to play by the rules of a system built on betrayal. Like Rowdy Girl, I was focused on saving the herd. She wasn't just fighting for her life; she was waking me up to fight for mine! The deeper I went into her world, the more I realized that I wasn't rescuing her, *she was rescuing me.*

The more I saw the world through her eyes, the more it brought into focus the truth and shattered all the normalized violence I grew up believing in. Through her I saw that killing her would be like killing me. Seeing the world through her eyes caused me to change *everything* about the way I believe. It shattered the walls I had built around my own heart. She pulled me out of tradition and into my *purpose*—one that I never saw coming. A cow! Rescuing me from the very last lie that love and slaughter could ever coexist. There was no way in hell I was gonna send her to slaughter.

So when some vegans came after me, I was hurt. I tried to show them who I am, and convince them of our intentions. I even invited them to come visit our ranch.

Finally, a wise friend told me, "Renée, haters are gonna hate."

Still, it took a toll. Tommy struggled with the hate more than I did. It wrecked him. That man is so good, and for him to be accused of being a scam artist just ate him up. He was consumed with the negative comments.

Keyboard warriors messaged hate around the clock and kept him up at night. Finally, I begged him to ignore it. But he couldn't stop.

Not only that, but Tommy was also shunned from the cattle ranching community. People would see him at the feed store and size him up and down. They'd have a conversation and interject snarky comments like—"I think they oughta take your Ag Exemption away from ya."

Tommy went from being an upstanding member of the Brazoria Cattlemen's Association to an outcast.

I never did this to be popular. If I wanted to be famous, I certainly wouldn't have chosen this journey!

I signed up for this because I knew I had to change the system. I had to put everything on the line. I had to remind myself of all the animals who couldn't speak up for themselves.

My mission was bigger than any critic could possibly understand. I had to stop trying to win them over.

Yep, converting from a bona fide Texas cattle ranch to a vegan sanctuary came with a few hateful vegans who believed I was trying to scam the vegan community and get rich quick. Those were some very nasty vegans, but luckily I had a deep spiritual practice. Because that's when my yogini came out.

The more people hated us, the deeper I went into my spiritual practice. I prayed for the haters. And the more they hated us, the more I prayed. Until finally, one fine day, all their bullshit was over.

Over the weeks, I would watch Tommy go through a whole series of emotions. Some days he was in total awe and was convinced we would succeed. Then, other days he would become cynical and depressed—not believing that we could pull this off.

Every day I was positioning him to talk to vegans who supported our fundraiser. Every day, Tommy's emotions were like a roller coaster. Some days he could imagine it. On other days, he was immobilized with fear of what it would all mean for him, his retirement, his family, and his position in the community.

As I mentioned earlier, Jeanne had recommended several documentaries for me to watch, and I was determined to show them to Tommy. I ordered everything she suggested, from *Cowspiracy*, *Forks Over Knives*, and *Vegucated* to *Peaceable Kingdom* and *Speciesism*. If I could get Tommy to watch these documentaries, that would be a significant step in the right direction.

As fate would have it, Tommy was willing to watch them all. He's a practical man, and he lives by statistics. Each documentary convinced him more and more that a plant-based diet made sense. He especially gravitated to the research about the China Study in the documentary *Forks Over Knives* because his dad had died of a massive heart attack at sixty-two shortly after retiring from Dow Chemical. Also, he found it extremely difficult to argue with Kip Andersen's statistics in *Cowspiracy* regarding climate change and the effect of animal agriculture on the planet.

Little by little, he was coming around. When he saw the donations rolling in, he was surprised, relieved, and shocked. He watched the figure grow and grow with pride and a lot of fear too.

Tommy would dodge other cattle ranchers in the feed store. His best friend and partner, Robert (God rest his soul), disowned him.

The *very same* Robert who introduced us at Michael's Club all those years ago before our first marriage, who had known Tommy since he was 18 years old, said he wanted *no part in that "vegan stuff."*

Everything Tommy stood for was deteriorating. Each day, something shifted inside of him because I was determined to go the distance no matter what. Whether showing him a documentary he always willingly watched or asking him to talk to another vegan, giving him a pep talk and encouraging him with love and support, he was always willing to meet me where I was in this crazy venture despite the odds.

It was like we were learning to communicate from ground zero. He went from having a wife that wanted nothing to do with the cows or the work it entailed to a wife that was frantic to do whatever it took to take care of them and keep them safe from the sale barn.

As the momentum of Rowdy Girl began to swirl around us, and around the country, our story attracted film producers, some legit and, once again, some not so legit. Through it all, Tommy and I kept taking care of the cows. We were consumed with figuring out how to sterilize the male calves and keep the bulls from breeding. It ain't easy slowing down a breeding machine to become a sterile operation when your whole business was a cow/calf operation.

Amid all the buzz of us becoming a sanctuary, Tommy became dedicated to figuring out the hard part of keeping the herd separated to avoid pregnancies. In the process, I got to watch him relax into the flow as he was finally able, for the first time, to get close to the cows he used to breed for profit. Instead of seeing them as a means to an end, he began to see them as friends. I'll never forget those moments watching him soften on his journey to becoming a compassionate vegan.

Watching the process Tommy went through is something I have a tough time articulating. It was a little like falling in love all over again. I would find myself in awe of him while we were going through this massive shift, not only *in our way* of being on the ranch but *in our way* of interacting with each other and the cows. Suddenly, I was a big help to him.

Before I went vegan, I couldn't care less about helping him on the ranch. Now, every cell in me wanted to do whatever I could to help him and the cows. Whether it was mending a fence, feeding, watering, opening gates, or whatever, I was down to learn and help. Tommy always wanted my help. We were working together.

Who knew that my going vegan would be the key to our future partnership!

A couple of months into the fundraiser, Jeanne told me about a contest held by Eric Day and Glen Scott Lacey, producers of the film *Vegan: Everyday Stories*. They wanted to feature four stories in the documentary. Jeanne encouraged me to enter. Tentatively, I checked the website, filled out the paperwork, and pressed send. A few days later, I received an email expressing interest in our story. A Zoom call was scheduled, and the next thing you know, we got word that they'd picked us to feature in the film.

Out of six hundred entries, they chose four, and we were one of them. As the news sank in, Tommy began smiling a little more. The reality of our cattle ranch becoming a vegan farm was starting to feel real for him. He couldn't believe the filmmakers chose our story. They arrived in Angleton, Texas, to film during our first *Vegan Awareness Festival and Fundraiser for Rowdy Girl Sanctuary.*

As our fundraising progressed, I decided to hold a festival on May 2, 2015, for one final push to raise the money needed to buy his herd. The donations had started to wane after hitting $26,000, and I needed $4,000 more to buy Tommy's herd and turn the cattle ranch into a nonprofit. Putting on special events was something I could do. I was accustomed to producing music and other events in the past when I was on the road with my band and as a realtor in Pearland.

The lineup of speakers included Kip Andersen. As you know, Tommy had become an avid documentary watcher and watched plenty of Kip's work. When I told him Kip was coming, he was stunned. I was mortified when I looked around the house and realized I had invited a respected vegan documentarian into a home with deer heads, animal skins, and a huge elk head on display.

I begged Tommy to take them off the walls and bury them outside so I could have a decent funeral for them, but he balked at me and laughed.

"How could I invite Kip into our home with dead heads all over the house," I asked.

"If he can't take me as I am, so be it. I'm not a vegan, and I'm not about to put on pretenses otherwise." Tommy said.

The only thing I could do was tell Kip beforehand so there wouldn't be any surprises. Just thinking of what I would say to him made my heart beat fast. What if he refused to be a speaker because we had a bunch of deer heads and an elk "heirloom" in our home?

After a few days of fretting over what I would say to Kip, I called my sponsor because I was obsessing and terrified he would think we were horrible people. After my call, she gave me a few reading and writing assignments and told me to get on my knees to pray and ask for God's help. I did what she said and prayed before calling him. It's funny how that works. Since getting truly sober, I'm finally convinced that I need help when gripped by fear, and I've learned to surrender, let go and let God. It always works, no matter what.

The conversation could not have been more positive. Kip was so kindhearted. He told me not to worry about it and that if we were going to inspire Tommy to see another way, we had to be compassionate vegans, even to a cattle rancher.

At this place in our fundraising adventure, Tommy's emotions were a roller coaster. I could see him changing but that change didn't come easy. Most days, he was excited and encouraged but now and then, everything would go black for him. He would become negative and fearful, and I would have to retreat to my spiritual practice and pray for him. Then, out of nowhere, his spirit would soar as the light of veganism slowly but surely infiltrated our home, hearts, and cattle ranch.

By the time the fundraiser arrived, so much excitement was in the air. Vendors were coming in to set up their tents. We rescued our first pig, Herman, from a kill shelter and he fit right in.

Herman was named after my daddy. Ironically. Herman was a lot like my daddy, he was scary-mean and hard to get to know. It took us a while to settle him down. Tommy was afraid for me to be out there with him, because he would rush you with big tusks and teeth.

I used to sing to him. I calmed the savage beast.

Daddy liked to hear me sing too, he was my greatest fan. Taking care of Herman helped me deal with unresolved daddy issues. When nobody was around, I'd talk to him just as if Daddy was right there. It helped me be with my daddy in a way that I wasn't able to before he died.

On the day of the fundraiser, I know Daddy would have been happy that I went vegan, and that we were on this path. He always said I was a chip off the ole block. He was a big dreamer, and he would have been proud to see me living my dream.

So here we were, $4,000 short of raising the money, our very first piggy rescue, and people donating to come visit us at Rowdy Girl for the first time. It was so exhilarating.

The speakers were all excited to share their vegan enthusiasm about a cattle ranch turning vegan in Texas, and Glenn and Eric, the documentarians, were here filming it all.

We had over one hundred people in attendance and raised over $36,000. Enough to buy my husband's herd and start Rowdy Girl Sanctuary.

Another monumental thing happened the day of the festival—Tommy went vegan. He said he didn't do it for the animals. He did it because *So Delicious Ice Cream*, *Follow Your Heart Cheese*, and *Follow Your Heart Mayo* gave him the reasons to go all the way in.

Secretly, I believe he did do it for the animals but couldn't admit it. It took him a couple of years to say he was an ethical vegan. However, now he is 100 percent an ethical vegan. He will even say that he's an "animal rights activist" occasionally.

It takes time to get things right. I literally had to shove veganism down Tommy's throat. I had to threaten him on more than one occasion. To his credit, he did talk to my vegan friends, asked questions, watched documentaries, and got involved.

The money and media coverage didn't come all at once either, we were only interested in the right kind of money and the right messaging. We didn't have to sacrifice our souls to build our sanctuary. We never would.

The documentary was fantastic, the complete opposite of our first filmmaking experience. Tommy got a lot off his chest, and it really showed us who we were and what we'd accomplished. The documentary, *Vegan: Everyday Stories*, became our snapshot in time that happened at just the right moment. It was a miracle that we were chosen to be included in that film.

Seeing our story on film made it all real. I thank my first vegan friend, Jeanne, for encouraging me to enter the film contest. She has no idea how much I love her and thank God daily for her influence. Thank you, Jeanne.

## Veggie Awards

In 2015, just months after CBS Evening News aired our story of going vegan on a Texas cattle ranch, *VegNews Magazine*—the most influential vegan lifestyle publication in the world—named me Rookie Activist of the Year in their prestigious Veggie Awards.

The announcement was made at the National Animal Rights Conference in Los Angeles, in a room packed with powerhouse activists and plant-based celebrities. I was seated at the same table as Moby, the iconic electronic musician and longtime vegan, and Jane Velez-Mitchell, a fearless journalist and unstoppable voice for justice—who's been one of my closest allies ever since.

That night, they played our CBS segment—now seen by millions—and I gave my first ever public speech about our transformation. When I finished, the room stood up. The standing ovation hit me like a tidal wave.

*Who knew that losing my mind on a cattle ranch would land me here—accepting a major award, shoulder to shoulder with legends of the movement?*

To be recognized so early on affirmed that the voice of Rowdy Girl was resonating far beyond Texas fences—reaching hearts, stirring change, and shaking the system.

# 19

# *Door Number Three*

*Going vegan has been the best thing ever for me, and my husband is gravitating toward the whole lifestyle more and more every day! He is looking forward to the sanctuary life. One day at a time, we keep putting one foot in front of the other. It just keeps falling into place because we have so many people out there supporting us! Thank you from the bottom of my heart.*

*February 16, 2015*

"God grant me the serenity to accept the things I cannot change, the courage to change the things I can, and the wisdom to know the difference."[1]

Those who know me know that I filter every waking moment, every breath, every step, every word, and every day through the Serenity Prayer and other spiritual lessons that I've learned in recovery from alcoholism. That prayer is the silver bullet to my silver lining. That prayer enabled me to come to grips with all the anger, hatred, and hostility I felt toward Tommy.

Tommy is the salt of the earth. He comes from a rich background, not in material wealth, but in family loyalty, kindness, and a genuine heart for doing the right thing. A handshake from Tommy is as good as gold in your pocket. His passions are tradition, history, artifacts, his dogs, and all things metal detecting.

However, before he crossed over the great vegan divide and slipped into what I like to call "door number three," he was an avid hunter and a staunch meat-eater like most male Texans. For Tommy to go vegan was a miracle.

Behind door number one is the *door of no remorse*—where suffering is hidden, and willful ignorance reigns free. *I love animals, but bacon though!* It's the default do-nothing door. It has to be shredded in order to move forward.

Then there's door number two, where the veil starts to lift. When people begin to see animals as friends not food. That trance is broken, and for a moment the lie may begin to unravel. Remorse may come in just for a minute. *Oh God, I would never eat Antonio the turkey, why would I eat turkey for Thanksgiving?* But no real transformation occurs. You keep going between door one and two, trying to numb it out. It's why I kept relapsing. I numbed it all out with alcohol and drugs—just like I had in times past.

Then there's door number three, *the door of moral alignment.* You turn away or go deeper. It's also where the heart begins to break wide open. Door number three, as I imagine it, is the vegan frontier. It's that unbelievable place where all of us who are vegan for the animals shed our carnist skin. Our very bodies are shocked by the reality of who we really are. We are revolted by tradition, family, culture, religion, and society at large that have turned us into animal flesh-eating monsters, just like vampires and zombies. We craved the blood of the beast. All of those cravings instantly cease in the world of door number three.

Not only that, but we also abhor it. We can't believe that we ever participated in such a world. How did we not see what was always in front of us? Well, not exactly in front of us but clothed in dark and stench, faraway places, so the reality of who we were and what we were eating would not be exposed. Instead of seeing the truth, we believed the fairy tales of "happy hens," "Milk Does a Body Good," and "free-range" cows, goats, and other critters.

When people enter door number three for their health, they see the world differently than ethical vegans like me. However, I don't care how you slip in. Just get here. Cross over that great vegan divide, and you will eventually see for yourself that door number one and door number two were just a bunch of bull shoved down your throat, literally to prop up a horrific and violent food system that exists to breed innocent farm animals for food, extreme torture, and brutal slaughter.

Being a vegan cattle rancher's wife with a husband that wasn't vegan was odd, strange, and downright painful. Living in door number three with a man hanging onto door number two with all his might was debilitating. I could see and feel his torment.

It was like spooky monsters hanging onto someone's soul, trying to keep them in darkness. I paraphrase Matthew 13:16, "Those that have eyes to see, let them see. Those that have ears to hear, let them hear." It was just like that. I could see and hear things I could never see and hear before in door number two. In that reality, we are plugged into Big Ag. Everything we do, say, and experience comes from the perspective they literally shove down our throats.

Big Ag is king behind door number two. Churches, schools, the media, families, etcetera prop it up. The roots go deep, ten thousand years or more. Big Ag fuels our entire reality with lies and deception. Every word and every move we make defends them because, if we unplug from the killing that is animal agriculture, we will surely die. That's really what we think.

We think that we have to eat animals to survive. We think that's where we should get our protein. We believe that God created animals to be our food. For real! Even though Jesus Himself was born in a barn with a bunch of farm animals all around to witness His birth, we still believe the lies. This fabricated bullshit is known as indoctrination.

No one is going to be waiting in line to get a barbecue sandwich in Heaven.

There isn't going to be any suffering in Heaven, so why would we want to participate in it on Earth?

In Matthew, Jesus taught us how to pray:

Our Father, who art in heaven,
hallowed be thy Name,
thy kingdom come,
thy will be done,
on earth as it is in heaven.
Give us this day our daily bread.
And forgive us our trespasses,
as we forgive those
who trespass against us.
And lead us not into temptation,
but deliver us from evil.

For thine is the kingdom,
and the power, and the glory,
for ever and ever.
Amen

Jesus didn't say, *give us this day our daily flesh.* He said *give us this day our daily bread.* And if we are praying to bring heaven down, then it's clear: if peace reigns supreme in Heaven then that means we are supposed to build it on earth. There's no bloodshed, no butchered bodies, no gnashing of teeth, no suffering. So then why do we allow it here, when we continue to pray for God's kingdom to come down? We are called to take care of God's Earth and everything and everyone on it. Why would we as good stewards justify slitting the throats of lambs or any other animals?

We don't need to eat animals. They are here to be with us, not for us. We can learn from each other.

I have come to the conclusion that there's meaning in the manager. The Savior of the world, Jesus Christ, was surrounded by sweet animals who witnessed His birth. I can't imagine he'd tell us, it's OK to eat them. Why would he do that?

When we save animals, it's a mirror of what Jesus would do.

Jesus left the ninety-nine sheep and went after the one. I don't think he got that sheep and then ate it! He didn't treat his lambs as food; he called them lost and loved them.

I believe when Jesus flipped those tables in the synagogue, it wasn't because they were selling cookies. He was angry about the buying and selling of animals for slaughter in the temple. He shut down commerce for a day.

Jesus always said, *I desire mercy not sacrifice.*

When I watched the documentary *Christspiracy*, I learned that the word *money-changers* in Hebrew in actuality translates to "violent-ones." I was shocked. I had to rewind that scene, and watch it over and over, just to take it all in.

I had always thought Jesus was angry because of the *buying and selling*, but Jesus calls them violent-ones. It's violence that enrages our Savior. And not just violence against man.

If you want to learn more about this, then go watch *Christspiracy*.[2]

When your church leaders, school boards, media conglomerates, and politicians are all beholden to animal agriculture either by family ties, business agreements, or otherwise, you have to know that *it* will do whatever *it* has to do to survive, even if that means an ethical vegan that just ran into door number three is ostracized by their family and their society. Yep, there ya have it.

Look, I get it—breaking generational curses that go all the way back to the book of Genesis ain't easy. But don't kid yourself, it's *damn* possible.

After Noah and the Flood, God told man that they could eat animals, but it was meant to be temporary. It wasn't a blessing; it was permission with restrictions.

But we pushed the limits anyway.

We've been pushing it from the very beginning. Since the *Fall*, when we reached for what wasn't ours. Since the *Flood*, when violence and corruption filled the earth.

Since the *Exodus*, when we were delivered from bondage but dragged Egypt with us in our hearts. We've been wandering—grumbling in the desert of our own making.

And then in Numbers 11, it all comes to a head. The people cried out for meat, even after manna from heaven. *And what does it say?*

> "While the meat was still between their teeth, before it was chewed, the wrath of the Lord was aroused..."
>
> (Numbers 11:33–34)

Craving killed them. They called that place Kibroth Hattaavah—*Graves of Craving.*

*How many graves have been dug because of our cravings?*

*How many innocent beings have been buried under the weight of our appetite?*

God never intended for us to keep falling into the pit of eating animals. It's time to get back to the garden. God always moves us toward Eden, not away from it.

I wanted to bring Tommy into the Garden with me. I wanted to shout, "Come on over to my side. The grass is greener, there's no bloodshed, and the animals can be our friends."

But I needed God to grant me the serenity to accept the things I could not change. That was Tommy before he was ready to become vegan. I asked God to give me the courage to change the things I could. That was me. Then, I asked God to give me the wisdom to know the difference. That was and still is all the truth that awaits non-vegans in door number three.

After my talk with Mr. Lyman, my attitude toward Tommy softly shifted. I started getting quiet around Tommy. I started practicing all the mindfulness techniques I had learned throughout my life. I practiced the yoga sutra from the ancient text *Yoga Sutras of Patanjali, yoga chitti, vritti, nirodaha,* which means when you can calm the mind's disturbances and brain waves, you are practicing yoga. In this highly volatile situation, I began mindfully practicing what I had taught and believed for many years.

It worked. I deliberately and consciously breathed goodness in and door number two out. Door number three is all there is!

Tommy and I, like most people in the world, lived behind Door Number Two—until I went vegan and dragged him through Door Number Three by the hair of his chinny-chin-chin. I'm joking. I didn't pull him through with force, but I lured him through, and he walked in all his own, just the same.

When he got here on the day I'd successfully raised $36,000 to buy the cows, he looked around and said, "Alright, whatcha got to eat?" When I cooked him his first vegan meal of organic quinoa, toasted pine nuts, and wilted kale, he hated it.

Blood and flesh are physiologically and psychologically addicting—just like drugs. Animal flesh is dense in fat, salt, and that umami flavor. It's addictive and lights up the brain's reward system. *Heme,* iron from the blood, can have a stimulant effect, and some people can feel an adrenaline effect after they eat a slab of meat. It dulls our intuition. It's not an act of peace.

Despite the addictive qualities of animal flesh, Tommy kept putting one foot in front of the other.

Truthfully, in the beginning, he didn't like my food half of the time. (And I'm a really good cook!) He loved my cooking when I was serving up deer cutlets or beef stew, but tofu and black rice? Not so much. However, he was determined to learn all about this "new plant-based way of life," as he called it, and started cooking more for himself.

Next thing ya know, Tommy is in the kitchen fixing up fried potatoes, beans, onions, jalapeños, pico de gallo, and tortillas. That became Tommy's staple. He lived on it for a couple of weeks while I experimented with other ways to appeal to a cattle rancher-gone-vegan's tastebuds.

When I think back on those tumultuous days of our relationship, I have to pinch myself to acknowledge how far he's come—how far *we've* come.

Tommy's favorite quote, the epitome of his vegan conversion:

*Veganism was shoved down my throat, I chewed it up, and I liked it.*

That's how Tommy fell into door number three. I kept cracking that door because I was all the way in. Finally, one day, he walked in and said, "OK. I'll do it for my health. I'll try out this way of life," and so he did.

The way Tommy and I transitioned from a Texas beef cattle ranch to a vegan farm sanctuary is rooted in so much more than life events everyone sees on the surface. It's the undercurrent of the experiences we went through as we were both catapulted in and out of different realities.

What eventually transitioned our cattle ranch into a vegan farm sanctuary was more than a business plan, which Tommy and I never had. It was more than a dream, which we also never had. It was an outpouring and expression of a revolutionary creation born when two souls finally came together at door number three.

We've walked through many different doors in my story. One was even shredded to pieces. But once we both walked through door number three, there was no going back.

We saw, for the first time, maybe, we could walk into the pasture and be friends with all twenty-nine of the cows, cows that were on the brink of death. Maybe, just maybe, we were about to give birth to an idea that neither knew we were pregnant with. This awakening, as I have come to experience it, was our spiritual child. We could never have human babies, but the God of my understanding had a bigger plan.

All I did was show up in door number three and completely surrender to God's will. The wisdom to know the difference has been believing in things I cannot see. Even though I had no idea where I was going, how I was gonna do it, where I was gonna get the money, or if Tommy and I would stay married, I kept moving forward, doing the next indicated thing every second of the day. I had to be true to myself.

Matthew 6:33 says, "Faith is the substance of things hoped for and the evidence of things not seen." I had all the hope in the world at this point. I was over my head in hope. What eventually materialized as Rowdy Girl Sanctuary is the evidence of things not seen.

I found myself praying and walking around the house singing that old classic by the Police: "every breath I take, every move I make." I felt like I was being reborn in the belly of God to do something that He wanted me to do, not what *I* wanted to do.

I didn't want to feel the pain anymore of babies going to slaughter while their mothers grieved for days. That was and still is my driving motivation—not to say that I didn't learn to want to do it for other reasons. As I went along in the birthing process of transitioning our beef cattle ranch into a vegan farm sanctuary, a whole different world emerged. It was like some magical castle in the clouds that was always there, but you can't visualize until you climb the beanstalk.

It was a strange experience to be moving forward with this impossible-seeming idea. However, that didn't matter. In my prayers, every single day, morning, noon, and night, I got the distinct message that God was in the driver's seat. The wisdom I sought was upon me, and all I had to do was let go and let God.

# 20

# *Who Hated on Us and Why?*

*Stand up for what you believe in even if you're standing alone because once someone sees you standing, they are more likely to follow. We won't stop until every animal is free!*

*November 21, 2017*

As Rowdy Girl Sanctuary began to gain international fame, haters started coming out of the woodwork. Remember us talking about those "unhinged vegans?" Yep, they were always there lurking, and ready to pounce at any moment. It was relentless.

After the festival, we began to get major traction and we attracted some major trolls. Print media, TV, documentaries, blogs, and social media rapaciously shared the news.

People on social media with fake pages began fabricating lies and distorting the truth. This symphony of hatred pulled our magic carpet right out from underneath us. Had it not been for my deep center and connection to God, I would have crumbled. But quitting was not an option.

The tale of a Texas woman standing her ground and forcing her husband's hand took root. With that momentum came extremists firing back in an attempt to shut us down.

In the beginning, I found myself consumed by the Facebook frenzy. I tried hard to counteract every single thread of vile comments. However, there was no way for me to keep up with it. What goes up sometimes comes crashing down. We started getting the wrong kind of momentum. As fervently as our supporters shared our truth and vision, the trolls shared untruth, chewed us up, and spat us out.

It was a horrible time, and we had no control. Had it not been such a massive part of our journey, I'd refuse to write about it because it was such a dark, painful moment in my life. I had never been truly hated before. They *hated* us.

Tommy had an especially hard time with all the bullshit. The hatred devoured him. Our friends tried to convince us to ignore them. I was able to put it out of my mind, but Tommy couldn't. He was glued to his phone all hours of the day and night.

At first, just like me, he tried to combat the madness. However, with every attempt came more hysteria. Like a dog to vomit, poor Tommy would return to the despicable comments. It consumed him. He would show me hideous posts, with pain in his eyes. "Look what they are doing now."

He'd show me doctored photos, memes, and outrageous captions about us.

"I can't look at that, Tommy. *Please.* You have got to stop looking at that crap. I literally do not want to participate."

The lies were boundless. They called us scam artists and opportunists. They said we were preying on the hearts of our vegan community for financial gain. They even said we weren't cattle ranchers.

It made my stomach hurt, and my back ache. I could not do what I needed to do to take care of these cows, to feed them, to fundraise, to pay the bills if I was wallowing around in self-pity about what some yo-yo keyboard warriors in God-knows-where said about us.

My honorable husband wanted to convince these trolls.

"If they could only see what we are doing, then they'll stop."

Of course that never happened. They were hell-bent on destroying us. They organized boycotts, and even tagged our sponsors, supporters, and donors in God-awful posts.

It was like walking through a minefield of headlines. Our names were plastered across the internet like the tabloids in the checkout line. Our story was twisted and distributed like pure gossip. Those tabloid stories appealed to the kind of trashy people who eat that stuff up.

The keyboard warriors took our beautiful story—one of love, healing, and transition—and they butchered it. It felt like we were targeted. We felt horrible that people who trusted us would also believe these lies.

But I knew my motives were right.

I don't even want to talk about these people at all. But it was such a significant chapter in our lives—the birth of Rowdy Girl Sanctuary being met with such adversity. I had to rise above it. I could not be on their level—on those low frequencies of hate, negativity, and death. I had to stay on higher frequencies—thinking about stories like Jesus and Martin Luther King Jr. in order to stay grounded and inspired at the same time.

I had to stay aligned with greater forces to bring this all about. I had to work the AA program with a fervor—having daily conversations with my sponsor about what it really meant to have a power greater than myself. I had to work the steps to stay aligned with my Higher Power, and remember: *my mission was greater than myself too.*

My mission was greater than, "my little plans and designs," as we say in the Big Book. Every time they'd fling mud, I'd have to keep rising. If you're going to make great changes, you have to take actions of great change. You have to make decisions based on the truth instead of fear. Over and over again. Every day. Step by step.

As upsetting as this chapter in our life was, while all this was going on all I could think about was the pain and suffering of the animals. I could picture them going through each step of the slaughterhouse—those horrendous images. The hate online paled in comparison to what the animals were going through—and the love I received from my new bovine family.

## Reflecting on My Why—My Inner Sanctum

When the world turned loud and more hateful by the minute, I found refuge not in all the senseless arguments, but in the stillness of the pastures, where the truth lives, unspoken, in the eyes of all the cows. There, in my inner sanctum, I returned to my why. Houdini, Magic, and Stella—the three daughters of Rowdy Girl—each carrying a piece of Rowdy Girl's spirit, and each one changing me in their own way, right alongside their momma, the queen of the herd.

Houdini is Rowdy Girl's firstborn daughter—and I proudly call her my granddaughter. I have her tattooed on my left arm, and I tell everyone she's family, because I helped raise her with her momma, side by side. Being part of her life—watching her nurse, stretch out in the sun, curl up next to Rowdy Girl without fear of being taken—was life-altering. In her, I saw everything this sanctuary stands for: continuity, connection, and the right to simply *be*. That bond carved something permanent in me. It brought my purpose down from the clouds and into the soil beneath my vegan cowgirl boots.

Magic, the second-born of Rowdy Girl, is especially fond of me—and quite the rebel. Once, she got out of our pastures and was roaming wild on a six-hundred-acre neighboring ranch. If not for the honorable ethics of a nearby rancher, Magic might've been loaded on a trailer and sold. But when I realized she was missing and called everyone I could think of, a photo came through—Magic, running free with a herd that wasn't hers. "Is this your girl?" he asked. And it was. Within hours, Rowdy Girl and Magic's siblings were racing to greet her and welcome her home. That was quite the scare.

Stella, the third-born, is another story entirely. Her daddy was Frosty, our longhorn, and she inherited every bit of his Longhorn sass. She knows how to use those horns to draw a boundary. Stella's a stunning beauty, and she prances like she knows it. She's bold like her momma—but unlike Rowdy Girl, Stella comes armed with them horns and a look that says, "don't test me."

Rowdy Girl herself isn't one to smother you with affection—but her love doesn't need to be loud. Her presence is pure electrical transmission. She doesn't speak in moos—she speaks in knowing glances, in the subtle ways she places herself between the herd and the world. Her messages go straight to my soul, bypassing language altogether, and she's chosen me to *be* her voice.

The way I see it, her family is my family. Love is love. Life is life. Kids are kids. God knew in His infinite wisdom that my destiny was to be the mother of Rowdy Girl, and together we would birth a revolution. All of this and all of them were worth fighting for! No hater could take away my "why"—my inner sanctum, where tornadoes, floods, and hurricanes could not reach. Nothing could disturb my inner sanctum. During the darkest night of my soul, I lived in this quiet, sacred place, gaining an unfathomable strength, determination, and the will to face another day.

In a culture where family is often confined to bloodlines and walls, my definition keeps growing. My Rowdy family and I are woven together, not just in body but in spirit. What we share will transcend our lives. The Rowdy Girl herd carries a sacred legacy that will live on long after I'm gone, whispering through generations, awakening hearts and opening minds that I'll never meet.

I'll never forget stepping outside the morning after the ranch became a sanctuary. The day before, it was still the Sonnen Ranch—full of cows destined for slaughter. But that morning, *everything* changed. Not the cows—*me*. I had gone vegan in my mind. And just like that, they were no longer food. They were my family. No wonder the haters were relentless—I had busted through the veil of denial, of tradition, of everything this culture tells us about who animals are and what they're worth. I wasn't supposed to wake up. I wasn't supposed to speak out. And I sure as hell wasn't supposed to love cows like they were my kin folk. But I did. And I still do. That kind of love threatens a system built on stone-cold silence.

And the backlash? It wasn't just noise—it was spiritual warfare. The kind that hits you where it hurts. That's when my sponsor, calm as ever, looked me in the eye and said,

"You're gonna have to pray for them."

I didn't want to. I wanted to scream. To retaliate. To prove them wrong. But she reminded me that resentment is the luxury of the spiritually bankrupt, and I wasn't willing to go broke over strangers on the internet.

So I did the only thing that made sense—I took to my knees, clenched my fists, and prayed like hell for the people who hated me most.

## A Prayer for the Haters

*Lord, when they come for me with lies, with hate, with twisted tongues—*
*raise me up in Your truth like a wildfire they can't contain.*
*No weapon formed against me will prevail (Isaiah 54:17)—*
*because I'm not standing alone; I'm standing in You.*

*Guard my heart from the poison of bitterness*
*and bridle my tongue from striking back—*
*not because I'm weak, but because I'm stronger than revenge.*

*Let me blaze with righteous boldness and burn with holy love.*
*I bless those who curse me—not to agree with them,*

*but to show them they never had the power to pull me into their darkness to begin with.*

*Create in me a heart too wild to hate (Psalm 51:10),*
*too clean to carry shame,*
*too rowdy to stay silent.*

*Let love be my weapon,*
*truth be my fire,*
*and You, God, be my anthem.*
*Amen.*

This mission was never about *me* being comfortable. It was about saving the cows and it was about *their* freedom. It was always about liberating them from humans that seek only to exploit and kill them. I had to stay clear, clean, and Higher Powered. So I had to keep praying *hard*!

Then I cleared the field. I stripped away the old lies, the bloodstained traditions, and every excuse that said, "This is just the way it is," and "It will never happen, Renée." I built this sanctuary with nothing but Texas grit, grace, and a gut-deep understanding. And I believed—with everything in me—that they would come. The people. The support. The momentum. Because it was the right thing to do. And because it was time for Texas to go vegan.

And that's why there's a Rowdy Girl Sanctuary leading the way.

Those times were some of our bleakest. However, I've always believed that during the darkest of times, great light and awakening are around the corner.

Wayne Dyer said, "When you change the way you look at things, the things you look at change."[1]

One day we had a cattle ranch. The next day, it was a sanctuary. And like I said, the cows never changed.

*But I did, and that changed everything.*

About a year after the Sanctuary opened, we were at our wits' end. We would have gone bankrupt had we not owned the land in Angleton outright. I was constantly fundraising to feed and care for the cows. Not only that, but the expenses for the tractors, taxes, and other repairs still came rolling in. Tommy's morale plummeted. Depression set in, and he was losing hope.

He was blaming me left and right for getting him into this mess with "crazy vegans" hating on us.

We were suspicious that animal ag was involved. We don't know it to be a fact, but every time we turned around, there were fake pages, fake profiles, and stalkers trying to scare us into giving up our mission to end the evils of animal agriculture. The speed and scale at which fake posts about us were proliferating online made me think it was a coordinated plot to destabilize our organization.

But out of the ashes, a phoenix rose.

One day out of the blue, there was an anonymous donor. They believed wholeheartedly in our mission, and they pledged to support us every step of the way. Suddenly, we had new tractors, money for staff, and other operational needs.

There is always going to be hate so long as we justify killing and consuming animals. My mission is to change that—to walk with animals not to trample on them. Of course, there's hatred in the world—but I don't focus on that shit! My recovery and my sobriety depend on me focusing on solutions.

Why would such a dark force try to dismantle something so rooted in love? That question stayed with me through the worst storm Rowdy Girl Sanctuary ever faced. It wasn't just a crisis—it was a test of faith, of mission, of my very soul. And strangely, it became one of the most sacred initiations of my life. And I am grateful for it today. It made me even rowdier!

When the smear campaigns hit—fake pages, fake profiles, wild rumors spreading like wildfire—I quit trying to defend Tommy and me against the noise of hatred. Instead, I got still. I lay down with the cows. I listened to the earth. I cried for every animal we once sent to slaughter, and I cried for the ones still trapped in the machine. That's when I knew—this was bigger than us. We were shaking the roots of a system built on blood, and the system was shaking back.

You see, animal agriculture isn't just about meat—it's about power. It's the backbone of capitalism. The very word *capital* comes from *capita*—Latin for "head," as in *heads of cattle*. Wealth has always been measured in bodies. In ownership. In control. That's why when a Texas cattle ranch goes vegan, it isn't just personal—it's political. It's spiritual. It's economic sabotage to a system that thrives on keeping beings owned, used, and silenced.

They didn't just come for us because we changed. They came for us because we told the truth—and truth like that disrupts profit.

But here's the kicker: the more they tried to erase us, the louder our story got. Our story had a life of its own, and no one could stop it. Other farmers started reaching out. Our inbox filled with confessions and quiet hopes and dreams of a better way. People saw us on TV, in documentaries, and they began to ask themselves: *What if there's another way?* And there is.

When you unplug from the machine, yes—it gets ugly. But it also gets real. And what we've built since then is more real than anything I've ever known.

We are not here to play nice with oppression. We are not here to beg for scraps of kindness from a system that feeds on suffering and heartbreak. We are here to burn the whole damn lie down and plant something honest in its place.

The compassion I have come to embody isn't weakness—it's full-blown rebellion. Rebellion with a pulse so strong it will be felt through eternity. It is the spark that scares the hell out of the killing machine.

Rowdy Girl is where Eden gets a second chance.

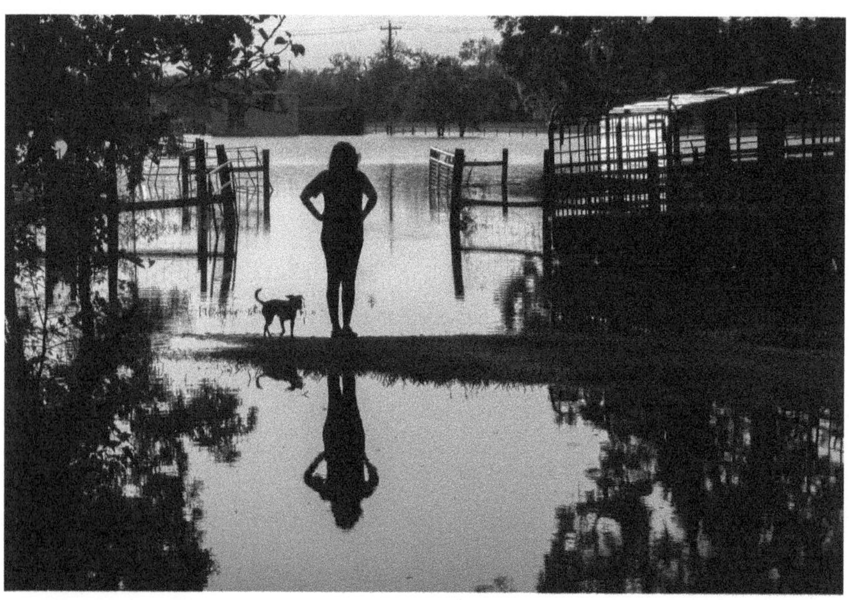

**Figure 8 Flood.** *The floods forced us to face the truth: the land that raised us couldn't keep us anymore. It pushed us toward the place where Rowdy Girl Sanctuary was meant to rise.*

# 21

# *Floods, Freezes, Heat Waves, and Droughts*

*Tommy and I often talk about the fact that we have always been in the middle of some kind of climate emergency since we started Rowdy Girl Sanctuary. When we moved to Waelder in Spring of 2019 we had been victims of three floods. Then a few months after we got settled in Waelder, the first wave of COVID19 blasted all of us. We had just gotten out from under the floods, massive disaster recovery efforts, the biggest move of our lives, and then COVID! And to compound it all the big Texas Arctic blast rolled in for two weeks in February of 2021 putting us all into another climate emergency.*

*August 1, 2022*

The first flood we experienced at Rowdy Girl Sanctuary was a hundred-year flood in June 2016. We had eighty-seven animals. When the catastrophic flood event began on June 4, we had no idea we would be in a state of panic, experiencing our first disaster recovery. The Brazos River started flooding over its banks, leaving us devastated and shocked.

This was a historic event, with the river cresting at its second-highest level ever, only exceeded by the 1913 flood. The ironic nature of this climate event is that it was not raining at Rowdy Girl Sanctuary. The sun was shining, yet doom was headed our way because of the rain pouring down along the dams and lakes north of Brazoria County.

The entire Brazos River Basin was inundated with rainfall in spring 2016. All the lakes and tributaries were full, and there was nowhere for the water authorities to channel the water. They had no other options, so they started releasing the overflow from the lakes. They knew they were releasing too much for the downstream communities to handle. They did it anyway.

The new construction upstream toward Houston and Sugarland had consumed the former pastures and rice fields, which were our safety net to prevent this type of water event. The water authorities had to make a choice. They had to flood Houston and Sugarland or the southern communities of Brazoria County along the Brazos River Basin. Some call this progress. I call it manmade climate change, greed, and overpopulation of humans.

All I could think of was the animals that we had worked so hard to rescue. Our chickens, cows, ducks, pigs, horses; what were we to do? How would we get them all to safety? There was no time to prepare. We couldn't even think about ourselves because we had to think about their safety first. We were in disaster mode.

Tommy was watching the weather reports around the clock. Our panic was immense, and it was hard to grasp what was happening and to know how we would respond. I felt powerless, but with that powerlessness came an innate instinct to pray, to depend on God, and ask Him to help us overcome this nightmare. When it was apparent that we had no choice but to evacuate, Tommy decided to stay behind with the dogs and the ground birds. I did not want to leave him, but he insisted.

We evacuated all the animals. Some of the animals went to the Brazoria County fairgrounds. Our main herd went to a neighboring pasture that was on higher ground, including my beloved baby, Stormy. This little calf, our blind Maine Anjou/Brangus, had a compromised immune system. She was a crossbreed we rescued from a breeder, and was like a daughter to me.

After safely evacuating all the large animals, Tommy insisted I take the cats and stay at his mother's house in Lake Jackson. So, Buddha, Melly, Shipaun, and I went to Effie's house. I took all my favorite novels and settled in for a long wait. Back home, Tommy never thought for a minute that the rising water would overtake the chicken and birdhouses. He never thought that the water would rise to the doorsteps of our home and leave no grass for the dogs to do their business.

As the waters began to consume our yard and it became clear that the birds were in peril, Tommy swam out to the birds' enclosures and began rescuing them all from drowning. He did this alone. I can't imagine the horror. Tommy has always been the survivor type, so if he were telling this story, he'd probably shrug and say he just did what needed to be done.

Tommy set up our adjacent garage with cages for our chickens, roosters, and ducks. Snakes and alligators swam along the front door. The flood waters kept rising. I decided to call in assistance from a Texas disaster relief organization and the National Guard. Tommy was hedged in with no way out. I thought he was a goner.

Lifeboats and big tankers mobilized. Tommy's sister, Lisa, and her husband, Elliott, and I awaited at the Buccee's on the corner of Highway 35 and 288. I was inconsolable. I broke down when I saw my family of birds, dogs, and husband, getting off the big tanker.

It was all so surreal. Our home, the animals' home, and all our pastures were under water. However, we were safe. This was the first of three flood events, each more intense than the last, filled with equal amounts of fear and disaster recovery preparations.

We took the birds and the dogs to the Brazoria County fairgrounds, where our pigs and loyal volunteers awaited. For several weeks, this became our headquarters, that and the pasture where our beloved Stormy perished after the flood, because pneumonia had settled in and killed her.

She died in my arms at Texas A&M in the food department. Stormy was our only casualty after the flood. She was like a daughter to me. To this day, I can hardly talk about her without tears welling up in my eyes and deep grief settling in on my heart. I loved her with all my being.

A love like that for animals I used to eat is not allowed in our culture. However, it's not only possible, but it's real, and it should be nurtured in our children, not driven down into insensitivity.

It took six weeks for the flood waters to subside. When we were finally able to go back home, we had no house to come home to. We bought an RV and lived there for ten months with, all the dogs and cats while our house was remodeled. We resumed our work and kept pace, thanks to many volunteers, donations, and angel supporters who believed in our work.

Another hardship came after Tommy's mother, Effie, took some falls and had become seriously ill. After months of caring for her, she passed away on May 24, 2017. Therefore, not only was I dealing with the grief and unsettling emotions of the Sonnen matriarch's passing, but I was about to be handed another catastrophic blow.

Little did we know that, one year later, after a total remodel and just getting back to business as usual, on August 17, 2017, Hurricane Harvey, a Category 4, would move in to destroy us yet again. It brought even more devastation because, this time, it was rising waters coupled with the fury of 140 mph winds.

We stayed at Effie's house again, only this time she wasn't there. Reliving these memories makes my heart, soul, and head hurt. We were climate change refugees again, staying in my recently departed mother-in-law's home. The emotions were almost too much to bear. On top of it all, I had to fundraise again to recover the losses and care for all the animals who depended solely on us for food, shelter, vet care, and love. Yes, love. Lots and lots of love.

Hurricane Harvey was classified as a five-hundred-year flood and was the most significant tropical cyclone rainfall event in Southeast Texas and United States history since reliable rainfall records began in the 1880s. Harvey dumped sixty inches of rain in Texas. Our home and pastures were destroyed again. The trees had lines of flood water measuring three to twelve feet, and all our fences were submerged in the flood waters. This time, we were displaced for forty days. It took us two years to recover.

We transported our animals again to the Brazoria County fairgrounds. One of our members, Michelle Cote, gave us a temporary home for our goats and dogs. Another neighboring sanctuary about 185 miles away cared for our herd and horses. We were again in a state of topsy-turvy madness, trying desperately to stay on top of all the sanctuary's administrative functions and payroll.

I remembered telling God that there was no way I could ever go through another disaster like 2016, but I learned not to tell God I won't be able to do something because sure enough, he'll show me I can. All things are possible with God. I just had to go deeper into the well of faith where my sanity could be restored second by second. I remember living between the seconds. The moments were too long. It was like I had PTSD.

Animal care became a round-the-clock job. I felt heartsick at being separated from our herd. They were two hours away, and I missed them terribly. We not only got through it, but we did so with unbelievable support from volunteers, donations, and growing followers.

These catastrophic events were horrible, but people showed up for us in the most astounding ways. There is always a silver lining if you look for one.

Animal farmers get unbelievable government aid when they raise animals for food. They get subsidies, insurance bailouts, and policies encouraging them to let their animals perish in the waters. That is the way of Big Ag. Just record your losses, and they'll take care of you and ensure you get another herd or a flock of "commodities" to get you going again. I couldn't imagine seeing our cows floating in the floodwaters and just cutting our losses. In our eyes, they were family, not food.

The perspective I gained while dealing such a tragic loss is immeasurable. I was so immersed in the experience that I couldn't process it all. I called my friend, Glenn Scott Lacey. If you remember, he's one of the directors of *Vegan: Everyday Stories*, which featured Tommy and me a couple of years prior. In less than forty-eight hours, Jon Meyer, a documentarian referred to us by Glenn, was at Effie's house and he followed our every move. The result was a thirty-minute documentary called *Ranch Rescue.*[1] He captured feelings, facial expressions, and the back breaking actions that it took to rescue the herd during the hurricane.

I never would have gotten through it without profound prayer, dedication to my sobriety, and deep acceptance that this was not being done to us *but through us.* This was an opportunity to prove the power of God through my willingness to surrender on a level that I never thought I could. God was indeed doing for me what I could not do for myself—*breathe.*

# 22

# *New Land*

*I love Tommy because he is a man of integrity who defends, cares for, and protects animals. He has taken the road less traveled, sacrificing social ease and even friendships because of it. He gets to love our animals without any hypocrisy or cognitive dissonance. He had a strong love for Sealy. He loved Sealy's feisty presence. When that turkey walked in, she owned the room! She was a beautiful creature who got to live out her life in our little ark in the middle of Texas.*

*November 23, 2023*

After the 2017 Hurricane Harvey flood, we knew we would have to move. We couldn't put ourselves, our animals, and our supporters through this again. We appealed to a foundation that believed in our mission. We made plans to start looking for land in Central Texas. We and our board of directors embarked upon a mission to find the perfect property for the new Rowdy Girl Sanctuary. We settled on 147 acres in Waelder, Texas, just 50 miles from Austin, 65 miles from San Antonio and 120 miles from Houston.

We signed the papers on April 30, 2019, and prepared to make plans for a methodical move to our new home. That wasn't to be the case at all. On May 15, 2019, we were flooded yet again. This time, instead of moving the animals to the fairgrounds, other pastures, etc., we prepared to move them all to the new Waelder location. The only problem was that the fences were practically nonexistent, and we had to crowd our sixty or more bovine family into closed-off quarters resembling a feedlot.

Frantically, I rushed to quarterback another disaster recovery fundraiser to help us get another $36,000 to fence the perimeter of our new property so that the cows could graze freely without roaming into nearby cattle ranches. We were surrounded by cattle ranches on every side, and the thought of our family getting mixed up with neighboring cattle bought and sold for slaughter was not an option.

As always, our amazing donors came to our rescue, and within days, one *single* donor donated the $36,000 needed to properly fence our new sanctuary location. The donor desires to remain anonymous, but suffice it to say, we call the two miles of perimeter enclosure "Emma's Fence."

Tommy had to move to Waelder to manage the current disaster and the animals. I had to stay behind in Angleton with the dogs, cats, and our prima donna turkey, Sealy.

Sealy was a *very* refined turkey. Her personality was majestic, and when she gave you a side-eye, you knew she was sizing you up; she either liked you or she didn't. And if she didn't, well, you'd know about it. But when she showed you love, it was pure and innocent. There was no denying Sealy.

Tommy and I were on the phone for hours every day, trying to manage both locations. The chickens had no coops and were in cages. Solving this became a top priority so our birds could freely express themselves without being confined.

Just thinking about these times gives me extreme anxiety. I remember going for a one-day visit and just crying over the fact that our once free-roaming birds that had secure coops to live in at night were now having to be fed and watered in cages. Their bedding had to be constantly changed with clean hay and shavings to keep them from living in their own excrement. We had to have fans in full force and ice in their water as the temperature was over one hundred degrees on many days.

Instantly, my mind raced to the Concentrated Animal Feeding Operation (CAFO) farm horror scenes I'd witnessed—birds crammed in cages without any care. The poultry industry is excruciatingly cruel, nothing but pure misery. The hens are forced to live in the same cages with sick, dying, and dead birds while being manipulated to lay eggs so people can enjoy a "balanced" breakfast.

"Renée, you best get back to the sanctuary in Angleton before dark," Tommy muttered. We were both exhausted. Trying to live between two locations was stressful. Being in Angleton without Tommy, the cows, pigs, horses, chickens, goats, and sheep was depressing. I cried every day. Sealy was very sick during this time, and I almost lost her. Had it not been for my dear friend, Sheryl, who lived next door to us then, I would not have been able to tube feed Sealy daily and give her a chance to live. Sheryl was a Registered Nurse and taught me how to tube-feed a turkey. She gave me the confidence to do it by myself eventually.

Sealy made it through, and I learned so much from Sheryl. Walking outside into the flooded waters with one of our dogs, Willie Bone (God rest his soul), was haunting. What was once our beautiful sanctuary was inundated with flood waters that forced us to become climate refugees once again.

I stared into a lake that was once our pasture with Willie Bone by my side. The fields that once were home to the Rowdy herd were again submerged by the forces of nature. How I got through the next few months was a miracle.

This chapter of my life was the toughest. Thank God for all my loyal supporters. Without the financial help, we would have gone under.

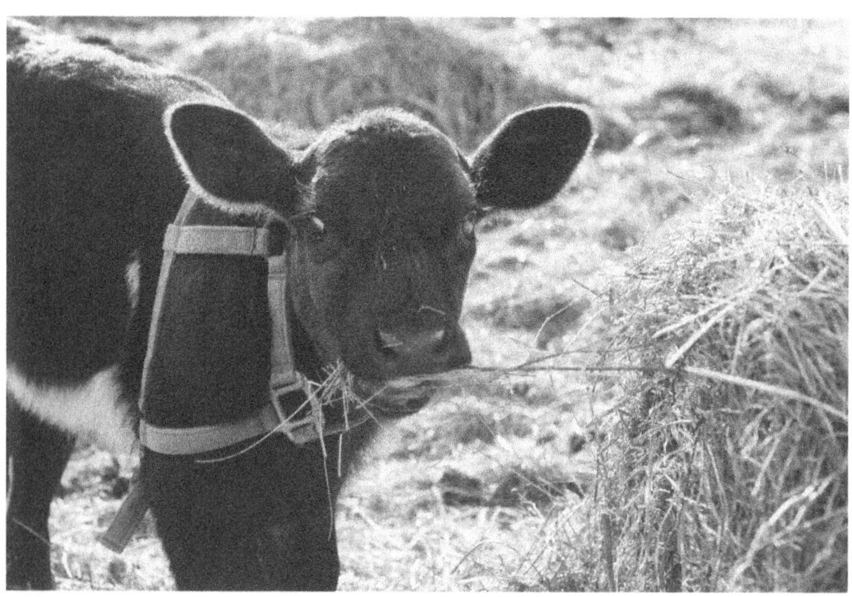

**Figure 9 Stormy**. *The baby who died in my arms at Texas A&M. Her loss became my vow: never again would a cow be treated as food by the doctors meant to heal them. That vow became the Medical Treatment Facility built in her name.*

# 23

# *Stormy's Medical Treatment Facility*

*In Memory of Stormy: Words cannot express the ache in my heart for my little Stormy Girl. Stormy was like the daughter I never had. I dedicated my life to her every single day in order to help her learn how to walk and navigate her little paddock.*

*December 14, 2021*

As cattle ranchers, Tommy and I considered cows as units of production in the food system. When we went vegan, they became our friends and family. They were all special to us. Some were extra special.

Stormy, our blind beautiful Maine Anjou/Brangus, like Rowdy Girl, was a daughter to me. Her prior owner surrendered her to us at three months old. She couldn't stand or walk for long periods, as her previous owner, fearing for her safety, confined her because she couldn't navigate the pastures. I dedicated my life to helping her learn how to walk and navigate her little paddock. I committed to working with Stormy for two hours daily. Every day, we went for walks so she could understand her parameters. We bonded fiercely and being her momma was the greatest honor. I bottle-fed, nurtured, and spoiled her with love, hugs, and kisses. Her scent still lingers on the tip of my nose. Hugging and nuzzling with her was like heaven to me. I was hers and she was mine.

This little heifer gave me and countless others nothing but love during her brief little life. She evacuated with the herd during the floods, and it killed me to be away from her. There was something sacred about earning the trust of such a vulnerable creature. She depended on me in a way no other animal had.

After the third storm, I was finally able to catch my breath and think about what happened back in 2017 at Texas A&M during Stormy's last few weeks on earth.

As you may recall, Stormy's immune system was weak and as a result, she caught pneumonia right after the 2016 flood subsided. After evacuating her, I did everything I could to get her the care she needed. She didn't have her little paddock to walk around in that she was used to. The area that we had to put her in was not nearly as big, and unfortunately, it was damp from all the flooding.

When she stopped eating, we knew she needed to see a vet. So, we drove hours to the Texas A&M veterinary hospital in Bryan College Station because we thought that would be the best solution for her. What I experienced at that vet hospital still gives me nightmares. It isn't the university's fault, it's the system's fault, but my little Stormy girl didn't stand a chance in that place.

For starters, they put her in the "food department." Stormy was a heifer, a living, breathing, beloved creature. Whenever I wanted to give her medication or treatment, they had to override their system. They were technically forbidden from using medications and treatments that would compromise the flesh of an animal considered food for human consumption. None of the vets or employees wanted to harm the animals, but they had procedures to follow, procedures that were developed in a system that doomed animals like Stormy from the beginning. I used my time there to try and show them how different the relationship between man and animal could be.

I told them I wouldn't pay them if they didn't take the words "food animal" off the $5,000 invoice. They told me that they couldn't change the system. I said, "Well, find someone who can if you want me to pay you." They did.

Every conversation I had with the staff was a chance to open their eyes to the cruelty of the food system and the kinder tenets of veganism. Since I was a former cattle rancher, the opportunity to make an impact was compounded. I hadn't started off any different than them. I was a Texas girl, raised on barbeque and rodeo.

I spared no expense to try to save Stormy's life, and while the staff were surprised by my efforts at first, the more time they spent around us, the more they understood. Despite many medical interventions and a failed blood transfusion, she couldn't pull through. With tears streaming down my eyes, I promised Stormy on the drive back, that I would one day build a medical facility in her name so that other beloved bovines like her would never be treated as food.

Stormy and her species are sentient beings with souls. They are not things. They have families and a will to live just like us. Sometimes, people don't believe it until they see it. Giving people the opportunity to see the complexity and compassion of these animals is exactly what we do at Rowdy Girl. I've invested tens of thousands of dollars in veterinary care, more often than I'd like, to no avail. I don't have a single regret. God did not ordain animals to be our food. Humans did that, and we can undo it.

I believe we are all born vegan—innocent and unwilling to harm. If you place a peach in one hand and a baby bunny in the other, a child will eat the peach and want to play with the bunny. It's only through conditioning that we're taught to eat animals, to deny the existence of their souls, and to uphold an industry built on exploitation. It's not instinct—it's indoctrination.

## Stormy's Promise Realized

Today, I'm proud to say that the promise I made to my darling Stormy is no longer just a dream—it's a living reality, unfolding in phases, each one represents a bold proclamation against the lie that farmed animals should be treated in "food" departments instead of given a standard of care that treats them as individuals, not commodities.

On January 4, 2023, we exceeded a $100,000 goal to build **Phase One** of Stormy's Medical Treatment Facility—a structure affectionately known as the Cow House. It now shelters our herd of over seventy cows through Texas heat, freezes, floods, and the everyday unpredictability of rural life. But it's more than just a shelter from the unpredictable weather—it's the beginning of a new model of care, one rooted in love, dignity, and the staunch belief that aging bovines deserve tenderness and respect just like us.

In **Phase Two**, we began laying down the bones of long-term infrastructure: a dependable road to the facility, a solar-powered water well, an irrigation system for our hay fields, and the extension of underground utilities to power what's coming next. Our team also began to grow—because buildings don't save lives, people do.

As we entered **Phase Three**, we focused inward—constructing medical stalls, outfitting a basic lab, and setting up office space for visiting and resident veterinarians who would one day come to serve animals not as commodities, but as patients.

Now, we're in the final stretch—**Phase Four**—a $250,000 campaign that will bring the full vision of Stormy's Medical Treatment Facility to life. With an anticipated $125,000 match, every dollar donated will double in impact. This phase launched in November of 2025 and will fund:

- a multipurpose bunkhouse with sleeping quarters, a conservative kitchen, and a space for educational gatherings;
- a state-of-the-art hydraulic squeeze chute designed to reduce stress and allow our farm animal residents to receive safe, ethical treatment;
- critical earthwork and culverts to ensure the land supports our growing medical footprint;
- staffing infrastructure, so our team can grow in strength alongside our vision;
- and the replenishment of hay and feed, because healing starts with dependable nourishment.

This project has garnered support not just from vegans, but from cattle ranchers too—men and women who, despite their professions, love animals deeply but often feel trapped in systems they don't know how to escape—and even if they did escape, what would they do instead? Their support reminds me that hearts can shift. That paradigms like animal agriculture education practices can be cracked open.

My long-term vision is clear: Stormy's facility will become a hub—a sanctuary within a sanctuary—where vegan and vegan-curious veterinarians can train, intern, and learn what it means to provide *heart-led care* for animals once labeled as "food." I want compassionate vet students to intern here, study here, and carry what they learn into the world.

But I also want good-hearted, conventional Texas vets—those raised in the culture of cattle—to walk through our gates and experience something different. I want them to witness what happens when care is not constrained by profit models or speciesism. To understand that medical excellence doesn't require a price tag on a life!

Stormy's Medical Treatment Facility will not just treat animals. It will transform the way we see them. We are building something the veterinary world has never fully imagined: a medical center for those the world has cast aside as food. A new standard of care. A new way forward.

Building these facilities has opened my mind to the future needs of farmed animals. My takeaway in all of this is that we are not just constructing facilities–we're constructing a future where reverence and compassion for farmed animals is the baseline, not the exception. And Stormy—whose life was short but whose impact will be infinite—is the heartbeat of it all.

Nearly everyone you ask will say they love animals, but *which* animals are they talking about? Not all are treated or even thought about equally. Even the smartest minds in animal science teach and learn in a system that gives privilege to some species and not others. It doesn't need to be this way; you can be loved by a dog or a cat or a horse or a bird or a cow. In my experience, the second you're loved by a cow, it'll change you.

# 24

# *When Cows Are Down*

*The battle is very real—it's a daily, minute-by-minute ordeal. Every day I get calls about animals in distress somewhere. Every day there are problems to be solved for the animals in our care. The clock ticks and my every waking moment now is spent on figuring out what, when, and how to do the "next right thing" for the voiceless. We all must rise to the occasion! We must put on our gear; we must be their warrior. They have no one else! If not you, who?*

*October 11, 2016*

The hardest thing in the world is watching a 1,400–1,500-pound friend down on the ground, seeing them struggling to stand in a broken body, while their mind and will to live are as strong as ever. I always feel so helpless and utterly defenseless.

When Sofie arrived, she came to us with an urgent request. Donna, her owner, couldn't care for her anymore because they were selling their land and had already begun taking down fences. The new owner told Donna to "get Sofie out of here, or she's going to the sale barn." Frantically, Donna contacted me, begging me to take her "right now."

Technically, we were at capacity. We always are. However, Donna's love for Sofie and her desperate plea propelled me into action. Two days later, she was here after a cattle rancher transporter kept her overnight at a sale barn until he could bring her to Rowdy Girl Sanctuary.

When Sofie arrived, she was distraught. She had lived her entire thirty-seven years in one place. Thirty-seven is unusually old for a cow. She was an old woman set in her ways, about to be offloaded into a brand-new world. Somehow, she lost one of her beautiful horns through transport and was bleeding. I can't imagine how painful that must have been for her.

She was wild-eyed, and as soon as the trailer door opened, she bolted out of the trailer and fell hard to her knees. Her right knee took the brunt of her weight, and had it not been for sheer adrenaline coursing through her veins, she would not have gotten up. Fired with unbridled fear, she forced herself up and skidded across the hard dirt. The ranchers who transported her were stunned to see her bolt up the way she did.

After that day, Sophie limped and walked slowly. It was difficult for her to get herself up, but she managed. One night, she couldn't get up. We all woke up afraid for the worst, but she was wide-eyed. It was obvious she had flailed through the night trying to get up. She was sweating and tired but not dying. I called the vet and put them on emergency visit standby. Lorianne, our lead animal caretaker at the time, Tommy, and I worked swiftly applying wide straps and using the tractor to hoist her up as we did with Big Bird (God rest his soul), a steer we lost the previous year. Big Bird gained another year by getting him up twice with straps and a tractor.

However, no matter how hard we tried to get Sofie up with the straps, her weight would not allow it without putting undue pressure on her. We tried for about forty-five minutes, gave up, and called the vet.

Large animal vets aren't trained to take care of bovines until the day they naturally die. When they come out here, or we go to their clinic with a large bovine, they learn a lot about true compassion for animals from us. In their world, they classify animals like Sofie as "food." It's as if, somehow, because humans have decided to eat their flesh, they should be treated differently and killed prematurely.

I always do everything in my power to give an animal like Sofie the chance to live if they have the will to live. I spare no expense. I cancel my plans and sit with them. I pray over them and send them love and light. I let them know that I'm here to support whatever decision they make as we do our very best to treat them as the individuals they are. We do for them what we would want done for ourselves. Sometimes, that means making an agonizing choice.

When the vet arrived, he did a couple of tests and determined that Sofie was septic. In his opinion, she was dying. The vet was willing to give her a chance by administering a boost of IV fluids, but in his professional opinion, it would probably not work. He was right. Halfway through the procedure, instead of getting the boost she needed to get herself up, she went into cardiac arrest and died. She didn't have the energy to get on her feet. She passed quickly. My big, beautiful Sofie was gone.

The realities and the ethics of sanctuary life come with real-world consequences. When you become caretakers of these majestic giants you have to make hard and complicated life-changing decisions for them.

One of those brutal decisions impacted Sydney and Terald, the last of our two regal bulls in our original herd.

Sydney and Terald were both intact and had lived peacefully in their own secluded pasture, separate from the cows at the sanctuary in Angleton, because we could not risk unplanned pregnancies. *Not at a sanctuary.* Not when lives are at stake. If we allowed reproduction here, we'd lose the capacity to rescue others still waiting for a chance at life. That is the catch-22 in this whole thing. We had to castrate Sydney and Terald before we moved them to Waelder. Making this decision broke my heart. It hurt more than I can say to make this call, and the weight of this decision still lingers.

Castration is not a choice we take lightly—far from it. But when you're rescuing animals bred into existence by an industry that treats them as units of production, there are no easy choices. The sheer number of farm animals on this planet—over eighty billion land animals each year—didn't happen naturally. That's more than ten animals for every single human being alive today.[1] This isn't the result of wild or balanced ecosystems; it's the outcome of human interference on a massive scale. We've done the unthinkable—we've manipulated their reproductive systems for profit, not preservation. And we do it over and over again with no thought at all of the consequences.

We don't believe in breeding the animals we rescue. It would go against everything sanctuary stands for—and would make it impossible to keep saying yes to others still in need. If we allowed the natural reproductive instincts of intact animals to unfold freely, we'd become a cog in the wheel of the very cycle we're trying to disrupt. Castration becomes a necessary intervention—not because we want to strip any being of their autonomy, but because we're trying to salvage what's left of it. It's a tragic irony—to save lives, we must interrupt the very life-giving act they've been exploited for. It's heartbreaking!

When we had to evacuate our sanctuary for the third time due to flooding and prepare for our move to Waelder, we were forced to round up Sydney and Terald and send them to Texas A&M for castration. It was the only way we could safely integrate them with our herd in the new location. Castration, when done properly, is not supposed to be fatal.

But something went terribly wrong. Despite every effort, both Sydney and Terald suffered greatly after the procedure. We brought them home, hoping for recovery, but their condition worsened. Never in a million years would I have imagined what came next.

Sydney and Terald passed away here at the sanctuary.

The veterinarians who came out did what they could, but it became painfully clear that the system they were trained in wasn't built for animals like ours.

Vet hospitals affiliated with major animal agriculture universities are, by design, also teaching institutions—where students are often involved in procedures under supervision. This model can be beneficial in many contexts, but it may not always meet the specific needs of animals like ours, who are no longer seen as livestock or "food," but as individuals deserving specialized care. Over the years, we've had many successful castrations performed on large bulls, and we had never witnessed this kind of suffering or inability to recover. It was devastating to watch—and to hope—and still lose them.

Most large animal veterinarians are deeply compassionate people—but they're trained in systems that treat farm animals as food commodities, not companion pets. In these systems, care is generally shaped by production standards, not long-term well-being. Bulls like Sydney and Terald are rarely seen for who they are—gentle beings, not commodities. Their deaths haunt me—not just because they were preventable, but because they expose the failures of a system that wasn't designed to serve animals who are no longer "profitable." *And because I used to be part of that system.*

I didn't choose this world. None of us did. But I'm trying to make better choices inside of it. And sometimes, those choices hurt like hell.

My point here is to elaborate on how important it is for us to have treatment facilities and equipment capable of giving animals proper medical care. Whether it's an emergency or standard procedures, animals deserve care on their terms.

It is imperative that animals like Sofie have care the moment they need it. Timing is everything. The longer large animals like Sofie are down, the harder it is to revive them and strengthen their resolve to live.

And then I think of Sydney and Terald, the last two intact bulls tucked away from the chaos of breeding, who would have gone to slaughter had I not gone vegan. Here's two bulls, beautiful and soulful, full of who they are—and when it came time to get them castrated, we had no choice but to rely on the system, and it failed them.

We had all the love in our heart. We had the passion, but we did not have the means. Love wasn't enough. We had the heart but not the tools.

This is exactly why we knew we had to create a medical treatment facility in memory of Stormy, the brave little soul who changed everything for us. Her death shattered us, but it also brought forth a vision—where animals like her and Sofie, Sydney, and Terald are honored and respected. Where excellent care for farm animals is the baseline. This vision isn't exclusive to Rowdy Girl, I hope other sanctuaries learn from us, and want to create a better standard of care for their animals too. Stormy's death wasn't in vain.

Every animal that passes at Rowdy Girl gives me a measure of power I didn't have before. Their lives bring me great blessings and much joy, and their deaths grieve me terribly. However, along with each passing, I'm gifted with their life as a memory in my DNA. Their memory gives me more power, courage, and perseverance to keep going for them.

After Sofie died, I posted what happened on my Instagram. Later, a follower shared this powerful insight on my post. It resonates deeply with many who believe that when we stop ingesting the energy of fear and violence, we begin to rise into a clearer consciousness. Whether through lived experience, energy work, or spiritual practice—so many of us know this shift is real:

> It takes thirty days without the energy of dead animal flesh for your consciousness to jump higher.[2] Their sheer terror from torture and murder

is in their bloodstream and bodies.[3] That energy attaches to our DNA and *becomes* us! So, we vibrate lower and don't have the consciousness we were born with. That is why you feel so different now. Since you don't have that energy in your cells anymore, you can *feel* more.[4] That's why more people need to give veganism a 30-day trial so that they can snap out of the robotic program. I'm so sorry for your loss. Sofie was beautiful. She took your love with her. Thank you for being there for her and all the other animals. God bless your farm.

I read those words and could feel them in my bones. I had studied this concept extensively, but I was grateful to be reminded of these powerful words while I was grieving. I needed to hear it. Sometimes we have to be reminded of what we already know.

Before Sofie took her last breath, I told the vet this: *I don't treat animals like food anymore. We just don't do that here.*

Every animal that I've lost leaves me a piece of their will to live. They have left a deeper call for me to rise in their memory, and for others like them who are trapped in the food system. The grief that I experience transmutes into a broader aspect of my vision.

Animals I used to eat changed me.

I carry all of them.

I carry their voice in my voice and in my fight for them.

They will always be with me, *always*. I never walk alone.

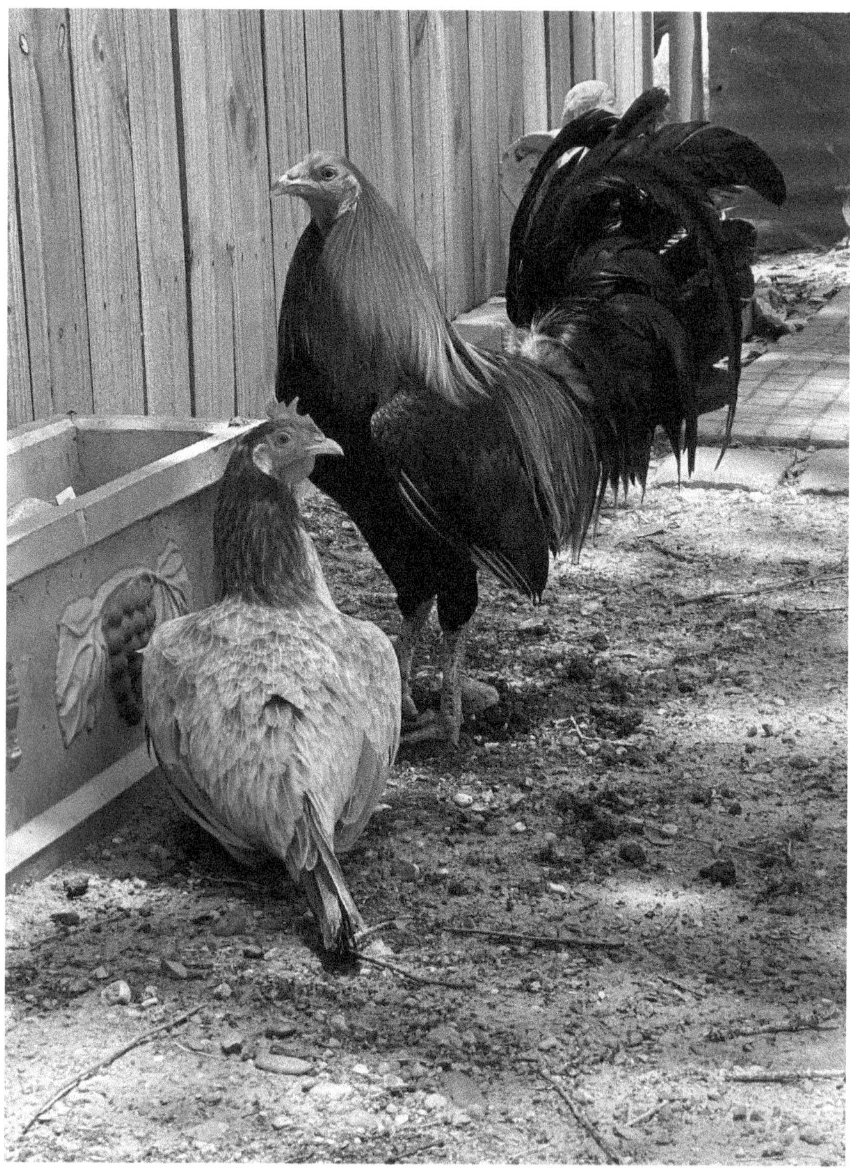

**Figure 10 Joaquin and Kiwi.** *Once victims of cockfighting, Joaquin was forced to fight and Kiwi was used as bait. At Rowdy Girl, they lived their remaining days as family, wrapped in safety, love, and freedom.*

# 25

# *I Love Chickens*

*Ain't nothing better than two chickens in my arms—pure love!*

*February 12, 2015*

At 7:45 a.m. on July 15, 2022, our sanctuary caretaker informed us that a raccoon had slaughtered and eaten our beloved chickens. Joaquin and Kiwi were two birds who came to us after getting caught up in illegal cockfighting rings in Texas. I stopped dead in my tracks. He knew the protocols. He had the checklists. At this point, our safety measures were proven to prevent such tragedies if implemented properly.

He'd made a mistake. The raccoons had left a crime scene, and our friends of seven years were gone. He resigned on the spot and felt terrible. My heart dropped from my chest and into my gut.

There's no way to explain my grief when I lose an animal species I used to eat. The grief is different from when I lose a cherished pet. Of course, I grieve the loss of my cats and dogs. They are family, too. But every time I lose a "food" animal, I'm reminded of the carelessness with which I used to treat them. I mourn for every creature I've ever consumed.

Throughout my career, I've spoken with many people curious about veganism who don't eat any meat, "except chicken." Chickens are loving, intelligent, sentient beings, just like any other animal you'd find at our Sanctuary.

They are deeply social. They can recognize over one hundred different individuals. They can dream.

Despite those characteristics, twenty-five million of them are just mercilessly killed every day. We've become desensitized to their suffering.

The unbearable pain of Kiwi and Joaquin's death reminded me of Dixie Chick, the first chick I ever loved.

Dixie Chick and her friends laid the best eggs. Before I went vegan, I raised her and a few others on the ranch to satisfy my craving for the excretions and fluids from a chicken's butt. Yep, today, I call it what it is. No magic curtain can hide the reality of the literal crap I called "food."

Dixie Chick loved to wander. I have pictures of her on our dirt roads in Angleton as an avid explorer. She was fearless. One evening, when it came time to put up the chickens, she was gone and nowhere to be found. I was terrified that a raccoon had gotten her. We had accounted for all the other girls, Dolly Parton, Miss Kitty, Lovely-Bo-Dovely, Twisted Sister, and Faith Hill. My heart ached.

At one point in our life, Tommy and I kept racoons for pets, but they were domesticated, and ate cat food and wieners. Raccoons, though cute and comical, can be vicious chicken predators. They lay in wait to devour their flesh and have the ability to penetrate deeply into their little bodies with their sharp fangs. Their tiny, human-like fingers can easily rip apart a chicken's limp carcass. I've seen it. I wish more than anything I hadn't.

Before we became a sanctuary, this was one of the horrors of daily living on our cattle ranch. We didn't have much in the way of security measures and it happened all the time. When one got picked off by a raccoon, it was just part of the food chain. We were sad for a minute then, we bought more baby chicks to raise so we could eat their eggs that, if fertilized (just like our infertile eggs), would become a baby.

As a new vegan, I took every measure to secure and batten down the hatches to keep Dixie Chick and the girls safe, but the raccoons were relentless. Once, a predator literally stuck its hand through a crack in the door of their coop and gnawed the head off a chicken's body. I felt terrible for all the other girls who had experienced their friend's horrific execution. When I couldn't find Dixie Chick, I was certain that a raccoon had taken her off for his supper.

Incredibly, a few days later, Dixie Chick came wandering through the woods on one of our dusty roads. I couldn't believe my eyes. She was limping, but she was alive. I yelled for Tommy to come out. How in the world did Dixie survive out in the woods where raccoons and coyotes were looking at every turn for their next meal?

I scooped Dixie up, went to the chicken coop to see about her leg, and got to work to relieve her distress and discomfort. In 1994, I got my massage therapy license. For years I practiced massage therapy and even had my own businesses. I let my license lapse after I became a Texas realtor, but my instincts to help and heal anyone in pain kicked in, and Dixie Chick became my first chicken patient.

I laid a clean towel on the kitchen counter and began to run warm water in the sink to soothe her injury. As I started to massage her little leg, I closed my eyes and felt every nuance of her anatomy. Slowly and with great care, I used my fingers and massage techniques to calm and ease her. She relaxed in my hands and responded positively to the tender touch. I felt the tight little muscle quiver in my fingers. I stopped, took a deep breath, and exhaled all the strain from her little leg.

Dixie looked up at me with her beautiful eyes, and my soul met hers. In an instant, I saw her, and she saw me. Her leg responded wonderfully to my hands as memories of chicken legs, wings, and breasts flashed into my consciousness.

"Oh my God," I gasped.

I used to eat these body parts with impunity, and here I was, melting into the awareness and soul of this trusting being.

As Dixie's massage session ended, I wrapped her little body in a warm towel, went into my living room, and held her. She snuggled into the recesses of my neck and purred like a cat. I wept. Deep waves of emotion flooded me. How could I eat a chicken's chopped-up body one day and tenderly use my hands to soothe one the next? The conditioning and program passed on to humans because of the corporate monster of animal agriculture is mind-blowing.

Bonding with Dixie was like something out of a fairy tale. So many fairy tales were written to awaken us—"Snow White," "Cinderella," *Alice in Wonderland*. I often use the analogy of going down the rabbit hole. I went down the rabbit hole and never returned. I had left the world of vampires and zombies for a place where the light shone, where animals and humans were kin. I used to crave dead bodies. I called it hot wings, scrambled eggs, bacon, or filet mignon. Now, I crave life.

May Joaquin and Kiwi's life always be remembered in the spirit that they lived. They were two birds caught up in illegal cockfighting rings in Texas. They were terrified when they were surrendered to us, but they grew to respect and live peacefully among us as family members. Rest in power and peace, my precious friends. I will keep retelling your story and see the world through your eyes.

# 26

# *Asha's Controversy*

*I never saw you, but I know you. I never touched you, but I felt you. I never met you, but I miss you. I know you're gone, but I won't forget you. Couldn't save you, but I fought for you. I am an animal defender and always will be.*

*—Maria Karlsson, Instagram post, June 22, 2023*

Navigating struggles between cattle ranchers and vegans is frustrating. We are all good people trying to do the right things for what we think are the right reasons. Usually, these two populations are like oil and water and do not mix well. That is why I have become a rancher advocate so that I can be a bridge between the two worlds.

Bringing vegans and cattle ranchers to the same living room is so important. Everyone needs to be heard, not yelled at. The situation at Asha's Sanctuary in Newfane, New York, in late July 2022 compelled me to seriously consider my views and how I would respond in the media. I didn't wish to piss off cattle ranchers, nor did I want vegans to think I was siding with the perceived enemy.

On August 2, 2022, Tracy Murphy, operator of Asha's Sanctuary, was arrested by the state police for refusing to return two cows who had wandered onto her sanctuary land. A local beef farmer claimed that the cows belonged to him and that her refusal to return them amounted to theft. Tracy maintained that the farmer had not presented evidence of ownership. The state police charged Tracy with third-degree grand larceny.

I'd watched the heated situation between Asha and the cattle ranchers unfold for several days. I was alerted of the controversy by someone who asked me to give my opinion in a news story. However, I didn't want to get in the middle of it at the time because it was so heated. I was immersed in the saga. It reminded me so much of my own old-fashioned Texas showdown with Tommy, a multigenerational cattle rancher husband with his family legacy on the line.

After the news story aired, cattle ranchers, their wives, and other family members started to contact me privately to talk about their feelings for some of the cows they sent to slaughter. I was overwhelmed with communication from all across the industry. I found myself having private, intimate conversations with folks that normally would never talk about "the feelings" they developed for animals destined for slaughter. When word got out about Asha's runaway cows, some of them were relieved. Even cattle ranchers have a heart for the cows. Once the cows are named and seen, some cattle ranchers' hearts can't help but open to them.

Who was right? The cattle rancher who perceives animals as "property," or the sanctuary founder who sees the cows as victims. Both sides have compelling arguments worthy of our attention. The cattle ranchers feared they were losing their identity. Animal rights activists argued that the cow's identities had never even been considered. The debate is as fiery today as ever, but it doesn't need to turn into an all-out war.

As a rancher turned vegan, I've made my decision: cows were never meant to be erased for profit. Communities were never meant to be split up. We should never have separated families, and sent their loved ones to slaughterhouses.

We were supposed to be good stewards, not play God. I empathize with cattle ranchers who are still breeding for profit—that was us. But when you know better, *you do better.*

When I looked at the cows who wandered into Asha's Sanctuary, I unequivocally voted to let them live. They found their way to freedom. Animals like these cows suffer every second of the day. No one sees their tears or the frantic look of fear in their eyes. No one hears their agonizing, guttural moans of despair and brokenness or the sounds of machines quickly hoisting their bodies, skinning them, sometimes while still alive and pregnant. No one sees their bodies dismembered while other scared beings fight frantically for what they know is coming. *They* see the sights, smell the blood and fear, and desperately want humans to have mercy. That mercy never comes. The last thing they see before receiving a bolt to the head is a slaughterhouse worker's eyes. These cows found their freedom. If they could speak, they'd have begged for their lives.

Matthew 9:13 states, "But go and learn what this means: 'I desire mercy, not sacrifice.'" This is a perfect opportunity for the ranching community to hear the voice of the humans that see animals as sentient and deserving of rights to their own life. Cows and all animals value their lives and the lives of their families.

Most vegans were not born vegan. We awaken. Ranchers are good people. Every single one I know is the salt of the earth. We do business with them every day and we are glad to have them as our friends and neighbors. I am an animal advocate *and* a rancher advocate.

I'm not here to condemn ranchers. I'm here to bridge the gap. The chasm is wide, but our common ground is our genuine, unadulterated humanity and ability to reason.

How can we make it easier for ranchers to make the change?

We all deserve to be heard. The cattle ranchers who support the local beef farmer in the Asha's Sanctuary controversy come from the perspective that someone had stolen their property. The vegans want to save the cows from slaughter because they don't believe an animal can be property. What can we own? Are our pets property? This is a whole debate within the vegan movement. That question alone could launch a thousand arguments. But to truly get to the root of the question, we need to get to the heart of the answer. *Do animals exist to soothe, serve, or save us? Is their reason for existence for us, or for themselves?*

For most vegans, the concept of any ownership of any sentient being is messed up. We don't believe animals are property, but it's complicated. We do live with our animals. Even as we rescue and love these animals, we are forced to reckon with the truth—that even our most cherished companions are still living in systems of control. Legally, they are still classified as property. That's why I can go to a pet store and buy an animal; they are seen as property.

So what can we own? If we believe animals are not here *for* us but *with* us, then the language of ownership begins to disintegrate. What if we saw them as persons with their own boundaries, desires, and agency? That's why going vegan challenges not just what's on your plate, but what's inside the whole paradigm of veganism. We are not here to be their god. We are here to liberate them, and sometimes that means liberating ourselves from the need to possess and control them. That's why it's so important to adopt and not shop!

The only way to approach complexity like this is with compassion. I always thought I was compassionate, but that compassion truly arrived when I became an ethical vegan. There are levels and depths of compassion that I didn't know I had until I started seeing the lives of animals through their eyes.

First and foremost, we are all animals. We are all someone. We all deserve respect. No one is a widget or a true commodity. These cows sought refuge, and even if they had never wandered onto a sanctuary, they would still deserve freedom.

Tracy Murphy of Asha's Farm Sanctuary was found innocent after a judge dismissed all charges in October 2024.[1]

*No one is born to suffer.*

*If we can prevent suffering, why wouldn't we?*

# 27

# *The Himalayan Vegan Festival*

*We've come a long way baby! In a little over two years our story has been told all over the country and in many parts of the world! Rowdy Girl Sanctuary is known as a revolution. We are known as pioneers—revolution? pioneers? I don't know about all that, but I do know that we are IN IT! The pace is indescribable. People come from all over the country to visit, to stay and to embrace our new life transitioning from a beef cattle ranch to a vegan farm sanctuary. When you are in the story you cannot see the story—the love and gratitude that is projected back to us is overwhelming at times.*

*May 7, 2017*

Nothing prepared me for the culture shock of Kathmandu. It was Saturday, September 10, 2022, at 6:15 a.m. The trip was twenty-two hours long, with a short layover in Istanbul. Leaving the sanctuary was traumatic for me. Honestly, I didn't want to go. However, my life had taken on new meaning since going vegan and creating a nonprofit. It had layered levels of service, plus a calling I never knew was pulling me. Veganism was a spiritual journey all on its own and I needed to understand more about who I was and what my purpose was in this new phase of life and learning. I was asked to speak at the Himalayan Vegan Festival in Nepal to share our story of transformation. It was an honor, and I was excited.

I walked into the dining room of the hotel where the festival was being held and saw Derek Sarno sitting alone on the couch, enjoying a cup of coffee. Derek cofounded Wicked Healthy, a plant-based food company, and is the director of plant-based innovation at Tesco (a major UK grocery chain). Anyway, my immersion into the culture of Kathmandu was made less shocking by the friendship and conversations I had with Derek.

I hoped to go to a nearby restaurant where he would teach chefs how to prepare his famous mushroom steaks.

At any rate, one of my goals was to go hang out in the streets alone. There are no sidewalks, and nobody cares what side of the road they drive on. There are stray dogs just lounging in the middle of the streets. Everyone sells anything and everything along the side of the cobblestone streets. The day before, as my driver sped past the storefronts, I couldn't take it all in. There were so many different shops.

To my dismay, juxtaposed beside the vibrant fruit stalls were markets where animals awaited their fate. It was gut-wrenching to witness—but essential. In America, the violence is hidden behind cellophane and supermarket walls. Here, it was exposed: limp bodies of once-living beings hung from hooks, while chickens crammed in cages blinked into the eyes of passing patrons, their throats moments from being slit. I felt the sting of global complicity—this wasn't just here, it was everywhere. The chaos of these streets echoed the quiet brutality of Western culture. And amid it all stood the birthplace of the Buddha, whose teachings of nonviolence seem forgotten in the shadows of every slaughterhouse, East and West.

For two of the four presentations in Kathmandu, I was paired with Mahatma Gandhi's relative by marriage, Maneka Gandhi. She had served in Parliament in India and was married to the late politician Sanjay Gandhi.

Maneka is a powerhouse in India. She's also a politician, animal rights activist, and environmentalist. After Kathmandu, we flew to Lumbini where we took in the energy of the monasteries and the wild surroundings of the culture. The third arm of the festival was in Pokhara at the Pokhara Grande Hotel, nestled near the beautiful mountains of Annapurna and on Phewa Lake.

The Nepalese people really know how to put on an event. This was their first vegan festival, seven days long and in three different cities! Their goal is to create a vegan community in the Himalayas.

I met many inspiring folks during my week in Kathmandu, such as Seth Tibbott of Tofurky, Ken Spector of Happy Cow, Sailesh Rao of Climate Healers, and Dolly Vyas Ahuja, director of The Land of Ahimsa.

I also met Emelia Leese, attorney and author of *Think Like a Vegan*, and Dr. Nandita Shah, an Indian homeopath, author, and founder of Sharan, a nonprofit dedicated to helping people heal themselves and the planet by connecting to animals and nature. Then there was Dr. Susianto Tseng, doctor of public health nutrition and president of the World Vegan Organization and Vegan Society of Indonesia, and Sebastian Joy, founding president of ProVeg International, a global food awareness organization with the mission to reduce the global consumption of animals by 50 percent by 2040. He's married to the final catalyst of my vegan transformation, Dr. Melanie Joy.

I met so many wonderful people. It felt miraculous that the Rowdy Girl story had traveled so far. I never dreamed it would land me in the Himalayas. It was humbling and exciting to be seated alongside so many people from all around the world that I admired so deeply. There were so many moments in my journey where I felt isolated, but the festival showed me just how big and how passionate the vegan community was. I was filled with optimism, the sense that systemic change was possible.

To say this experience changed me is an understatement. Witnessing the breathtaking beauty, complexity, and suffering in the streets left an imprint I'll carry for the rest of my life. It shaped my values and ignited my fight.

We are one people, one planet, one truth. There really is no border outside the physical confines of our imagined ownership of Mother Earth, the mother we all need and share. We are Earthlings. I've heard this time and time again. However, just like I used to eat animals and think I loved them, I have also claimed to be an Earthling with no concept of the other side of the Earth until Kathmandu.

As a former Texas cattle rancher, I harbored many secrets. As I stared into the distance at Pokhara's beautiful Annapurna mountains, these secrets boldly came to life as I witnessed my mind's awakening. Raised Christian, I was taught that Christianity was the only way to heaven. Yet here I am in one of the many mansions Christ spoke of in the Bible. "In my Father's house, there are many mansions: if it were not so, I would have told you. I go to prepare a place for you." (2 Timothy 2:15)

Those many mansions are yet another doorway in my consciousness that Christ has prepared for me, ready for when I'm able to walk through and trust that He is there to welcome my next awakening. It's time that we all put our preconceived notions aside about who we think we are. That includes the program that taught us we were separate from animals. We've never been separate!

Only through culture, which God did not create, is it hammered into our individual consciousness to bow to the God, tradition, and culture we're born into. Otherwise, we would surely face certain death, ostracization from our families, and exile from our respective countries. We would be traitors to the dogma and program holding the power structure of our individual and collective belief systems together. Those systems are like the glue that prevents us from merging into the oneness that is our true birthright.

The Jesus I serve, and love was not a Christian. He was a Jew. I don't believe for a minute that He ever intended to create a consciousness in Christians that was so dogmatic, self-serving, and innately cruel to animals.

The foundation of our world has been laid on the broken bodies of meek animals. We've made ourselves rulers of a kingdom that was never ours to claim.

That's the work of human domination, rather than Divine Design.

*We've mistaken Dominion for absolute destruction.*

The Bible says to "study to show yourself approved" (2 Timothy 2:15), and "seek and you shall find" (Matthew 7:7). I have studied, and I have searched, and I found the truth as I know it through the eyes of a *vegan Christian.*

If we pull out of that paradigm where we serve beliefs instead of the *one* Creator that created us all, we will walk through into another mansion promised to us by Christ Himself.

Consider this verse from Ecclesiastes 3:19. "For what happens to the sons of men also happens to animals; one thing befalls them: as one dies, so dies the other. Surely, they all have *one* breath; man has *no advantage* over animals, for all is vanity."

The Jesus I have come to know loves the Jews, Buddhists, Muslims, Hindus, Taoists, Sikhs, and all. Only *we*, with our cultured backgrounds, family origins, and tiring traditions, have invented borders, boundaries, and beliefs that only serve to perpetuate separation. This must indeed grieve the Father that created all of us.

God wanted us to share in the bounty and beauty of Mother Earth. He wanted us to learn from the master teachers, not create self-serving dogma. As a former cattle rancher, when I stepped into the world of veganism, the mansion of animal rights and ethics awaited me. I promise you—it's there for all of us.

Coming to the Himalayas to spend time with so many people from around the world has broadened my understanding and scope further. My prayer was that, as I journeyed back home to the Texas heartbeat of Rowdy Girl Sanctuary, I would cherish yet another secret—this new mansion given to me as I gazed upon the Annapurna mountains.

From these heights, I could clearly see the devastation and madness our people have created. Our planet is on fire. We've heated up real good, and now it's time for us all to become not only climate healers but animal healers.

We must do everything in our personal power to heal Mother Earth, who is crying because all her kids are screaming at each other. They are killing each other and killing other species in the name of "food," "clothing," "entertainment," and "experiments." We must stop the burning of our Earth and let go of our conditioning. We need to enter the mansion waiting for us all, where true compassion for all beings is the norm. It's time to exit our respective cultures that normalize violence.

I crave a vegan world. If a vegan cattle rancher can go around the planet and still find another mansion, so can you. Let's leave the confines of our glued boundaries and beliefs. There is always another awakening. We can rid ourselves of the archaic and barbaric beliefs that animals were created to be our food.

What truly transformed me during my time in Nepal wasn't just the conference—it was the people, the energy, and the soul of the place. The Buddhist monks moved with such presence and stillness, their very being was a lesson. Their peaceful discipline and reverence for all life softened something in me.

I made friendships that continue to shape me—one in particular was Emilia Leese, a fellow author and radiant soul whose kindness and clarity grounded me more than once. Another was Derek Sarno, who gave me the courage to step into the chaos of Kathmandu's streets with wide eyes and an open heart.

Being with my dear friends Dr. Sailesh Rao, founder of Climate Healers and executive producer of so many powerful documentaries, and Dolly Ahuja, the filmmaker behind *The Land of Ahimsa*, deepened my sense of purpose. Our shared mission—to end the suffering of animals—felt even more alive, more sacred, in that place. Together, we dreamed big, cried a little, and stood rooted in our collective vow to birth a vegan world.

And then there were the monkeys. During one of our group meditations, they surrounded us—not as distractions, but as participants. They sat with us, moved with us, and reminded me that the sacred circle includes all beings. The music and dancing, too, weren't performative. They were innocent, raw, full of heart—a reflection of community in its purest form. I could've stayed in those gardens for days. They were exquisite, like the spirit of Nepal itself.

We all sometimes need a geographical break to soar to new heights. I had no idea my trip to the Himalayas would yield such fruit. Oh, and the fruit! It was like nectar! I could make a whole meal with papaya and melons. I miss the sweetness, but so much of it lingers in my soul. The beautiful Nepalese people will forever dance and sing in my heart.

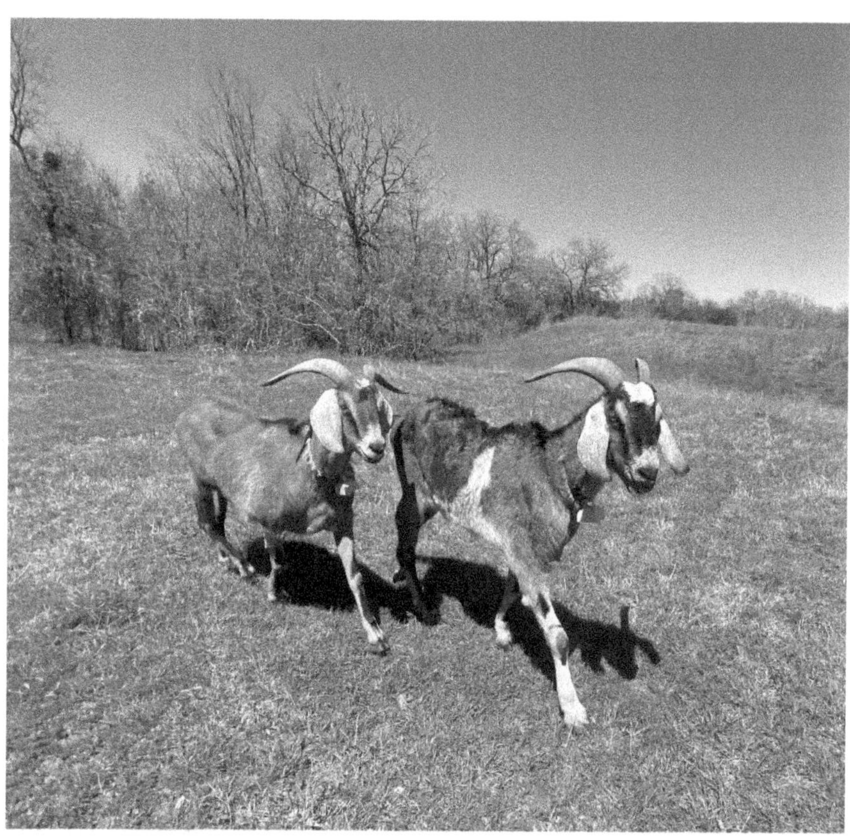

**Figure 11 Danny and Doogie.** *Inseparable brothers, each with his own spirit: Doogie was the fearless leader. Danny was the calm and tender heart who never left his side.*

# 28

# *A Tribute to Doogie and Danny*

*Doogie is now with Danny over the rainbow bridge! There is nothing easy about losing animals you grow to love in a sanctuary. A new level of compassion opened up in my heart the day I surrendered to my vegan heart. I never knew I had the capacity for so much empathy before going vegan! Thank you Doogie for being such a supermodel of pure love and for teaching Tommy and I to love even more. Your spirits will now merge with my own and will make me a stronger voice for God's creation!*

*January 12, 2023*

Doogie and his brother Danny were born in March 2011. They were inseparable. An elderly couple, who had the two brothers since birth, surrendered them to us on March 13, 2022. They could no longer care for Doogie and Danny because they were moving north to Vermont to be with their family and didn't want the bonded pair to end up slaughtered in the food system.

We knew when we said yes to these two that we would be in for heartbreak sooner rather than later. Doogie and Danny had never been around other goats, and they walked in tandem as if they were one body. Danny was Doogie's shadow. When Doogie walked, Danny followed. Doogie was outgoing while Danny was the gentle and shy soul. Seeing the two of them together made my heart swell with joy, knowing we could give them this opportunity to thrive in their elder years.

Tommy said they were like two old men. *Best friends.*

On June 12, 2022, the temperatures soared quickly and scorched Texas with one of the hottest days on record. Heat bursts can cause temperatures to spike quickly which can lead to dehydration, heat stress, and even collapse. Temperatures raged to 110 degrees Fahrenheit.

We had to work harder than ever to provide more shade, fans, frozen water, and extra hydration for our animals. Our older animals with special needs are always the most vulnerable.

Poor Danny was one of the affected animals—he collapsed. Even with extreme temperature protocols, and all our safety measures in place, we couldn't work fast enough to revive him.

Danny passed away from heat stroke.

Poor Doogie was lost without his best friend. He bellowed and cried for his friend. I had to lie down and console him.

"I'm here for you," I'd say. "We're not going anywhere."

We became his people.

After Danny died, Doogie didn't want to be with anybody but us—not even the other goats. He wanted nothing to do with them. Heck he probably didn't even know he was a goat.

He would walk into my office, like he owned the place. *And he did.*

We'd hear his little bell jingling and just smile and think, "Well here comes Doogie."

They say dogs are a man's best friend, but this goat would give any dog a run for its money. He was joined at the hip with Tommy. Whenever Tommy walked out of the office, or worked on the farm, Doogie would follow him everywhere.

Doogie was the kind of friend with a look in his eyes that told you he was aware of everything happening around him. He would hang out on the front porch like he was on a surveillance team. You could tell he was in a whole different world.

I would habitually take all my banana peels over to Doogie because that was his favorite snack. He couldn't eat them fast enough! That boy could devour a bag of greens like nobody's business.

Doogie and Tommy became great friends. Next to Murray, a grand Holstein that passed away in 2019 after our move to Waelder, Doogie is right up there inside Tommy's most tender of places in his vegan heart. Despite being a former cattle rancher, my husband has broken free from the animal production mentality. He is now wide open to experiencing all the love he is capable of for the animals he would have normally slaughtered in our food system.

Despite losing Danny, Doogie thrived. He was a super goat and was almost 13 when he passed away peacefully on January 11, 2023, of old age.

Eight to ten is old for a goat, and 13 is a good long life—but still, there is nothing easy about losing animals you grow to love in a sanctuary.

Tommy gets the harrowing job of burying all our animals when they die, which is extremely hard on him.

*Thought experiment:* Imagine what it would be like if every rancher and animal farmer were required to bury the animals they kill for food, not as waste but as lives once lived, just like a family pet. Could they still call them food products? Could they still call it "feeding the world"?

What might shift if just once they had to lay down the bodies of the animals they raise for food with dignity?

Perhaps it's in the burying not the butchering that we begin to reclaim our lost humanity.

*Thank you, Doogie and Danny, for being such supermodels of pure love and character and teaching Tommy and me to love harder. I love you both so much and will miss you and the sound of your Rowdy Girl bells.*

*Doogie, I will especially miss your passion for banana peels, your slipping into my office, and that quirky, knowing smile and eyes full of wisdom. Seeds of your spirits will now merge with my own and make me a stronger voice for God's creation. Until we meet again, my friends*

# 29

# *My First ThanksLiving*

*I'm getting to the point where I can hardly stand to even go to the grocery store. Tonight while at HEB I was in tears looking at the freezers with "young" turkeys boldly promoted as a "good" thing. Turkeys are fed enormous amounts of food after they are hatched. They yearn to find their mother and are scared and confused.*

*November 10, 2015*

You gain an awful lot when you become vegan, but you can lose a lot too. At least, it can feel that way. Veganism is countercultural. Much like sobriety, veganism can affect the way we interact with celebration, togetherness, and tradition. The good news is that it also gives us the opportunity to reinvent tradition.

Thanksgiving 2014 was extremely stressful. It was my first as a vegan. The thought of being around an entire turkey bird in the middle of the family table made me terribly sad.

I broke down in tears when I saw it, and the mood remained tense for the entire meal. When I saw the remains of the turkey bones in the sink after everyone had taken every shred of flesh for leftovers, it made me so sick that we had to leave.

Before my breakdown, I would have been standing around the island in the kitchen helping clean up, putting leftovers in a bowl for turkey sandwiches and salad. The room would feel warm, full of the holiday spirit. I loved being with my family, but I didn't know how to do it anymore. I worried I would never be able to participate in the holiday gatherings again. I wanted to feel included, part of the celebration, but my feelings for the animals they were eating consumed me.

But now, all I can see are my two precious turkeys, Chi Chi and Alana, whom we rescued from a 4-H family in 2016.

That day, we had seen a flyer in a health food store advertising turkeys for sale for $50 each.

At the time, we had two documentarians from Australia who came across the world to film our sanctuary—Chee Wei Tay from De Claffer films, and Alana Tompson from Black Ant Films.

"You could call her," Chee Wei nudged me.

"OK," I said without hesitation.

I called the number and asked the breeder, named Lillie, who said she would be willing to pardon two turkeys. Just like the president does every Thanksgiving.

Lillie asked why we were interested, and I told her our story.

To our relief, she agreed! We were elated.

Chee Wei and Alana filmed Tommy and me as we headed to the turkey breeder's farm. Lillie's kids were in the Future Farmers of America (FFA) about to wrap up their semester.

FFA is a student organization that trains youth in agriculture, leadership, and career paths—including how to farm animals for food. They're treated as meat from day one, but those who truly love animals choose not to participate in the violence at all. But sometimes kids and families get caught up in FFA, not knowing what is going to happen at the end of the day. Rowdy Girl Sanctuary is home to forty-plus animals who ended up at our sanctuary just this way.

Many students have no idea until the end comes that their friend is going to be slaughtered. They don't realize until it's too late that "their project" ends in heartbreak. They fall in love with a friend, only to be told that the friend is now going to be butchered. That's how the desensitization begins, because they feel forced to comply with the roles of education.

We went out to Lillie's farm and met our two new feathered friends. I wondered why she chose these two out of all of the turkeys in the cages. I can't tell the story of those other eighteen birds—other than they were eaten by families just like mine and yours.

Lillie kindly opened her heart to us, and I hugged her as she gently released the two fluffy white turkeys from the pen. They were just babies—still peeping, still soft, still trusting. Most people don't realize that the vast majority of turkeys slaughtered for food are only 12 to 15 weeks old.

*Poults*—that's what they're called at that age.

Not even old enough to really know the world, but old enough to be taken from it.

All of their friends were processed, slaughtered, sitting in a freezer somewhere, waiting for the final curtain call to be the centerpiece on an American table somewhere to be eaten.

*As is tradition.*

We named the turkeys Alana and Chi Chi after our incredible documentarians who captured the rescue on camera.

The documentary, called *The Rescue*, went on to win bronze at the Fiftieth WorldFest, Houston International Film Festival.

But the best prize for us was getting to extend the life of these two incredible birds.

Every year, close to forty-six million turkeys are slaughtered for Thanksgiving alone. That equates to 3,833,333 turkeys a month, 884,615 turkeys per week, or 126,373 turkeys daily.[1] That's 5,266 turkeys killed every hour of the day for Americans to celebrate Thanksgiving![2]

All we've done is create a commodity out of a living being on a holiday we probably shouldn't be celebrating anyway.

It's a way for businesses to drive up their numbers every year because they know people like you and me want to spend time with family. They know that people like us honor traditions and value special moments and we're willing to shell out the money to do it.

My dear friend and mentor, Dr. Sailesh Rao, often says we're not just farming animals—we're being farmed ourselves.[3] These systems, born from colonialism, were designed to condition us into consuming violence—against animals, the Earth, and each other. We've become cogs in a machine that feeds off our health, our hearts, and our humanity.[4] Once I understood that, I couldn't play along anymore.

Animal agriculture is farming humans to eat the animals they produce by literally forcing "Big Ag ideology" and *cult*ure down our throats. It's so pervasive that when a new vegan tells their family they will no longer eat turkey at the traditional Thanksgiving holiday, the family members think there's something wrong with them. Often, the vegan thinks there's something wrong with them too.

There's nothing wrong with making kindness and compassion the foundation for our food choices instead of violence and there's no reason other than clever marketing campaigns and conditioning that we can't take part in the traditions we love. Heck, we can make them better!

The thought of a family praying over turkeys as a celebratory meal while family members dismember their roasted bodies was all I could imagine. Why had I never seen, felt, or realized the pain and agony these smart and intelligent beings endure just to be someone's *Thanksgiving* every year?

It took me years to question the story of Thanksgiving. I grew up thinking it was a day of gratitude and tradition. But behind the feel-good narrative is a darker reality—both for Indigenous peoples and for animals. The holiday whitewashes colonization and celebrates a violent history with a feast built on the bodies of animals who never wanted to die. Once I saw that, I couldn't unsee it. Gratitude means more when it doesn't come at the cost of someone else's life.

And that's why I call it "Thanks*Living*" today.

The first time I heard the term *ThanksLiving*, it all clicked. It wasn't just a clever play on words—it was a complete reimagining of what it means to give thanks. That year, I celebrated with Cooper, a turkey we had rescued from the fate so many others face. Cooper came to us from one of our members named Michael Cooper and Lizzy Hargrove. They bought the poult from a feed store, and he needed a home ASAP.

That first *ThanksLiving*, we honored his life. We laid out a beautiful tray filled with pureed pumpkin, blueberries, cranberries, and grapes—foods that smelled like the season but didn't require suffering.

I watched Cooper gently peck at the feast we made just for him, and I felt something shift deep in my soul. This was what Thanksgiving was always supposed to be about—not tradition rooted in violence, but love rooted in presence.

So many families bow their heads and give thanks for the so-called food on their plates—birds like Chi Chi, Alana, and Cooper. But I could never give thanks for their dead bodies.

On *ThanksLiving*, we do something radically different. We give thanks for the lives of the turkeys who have found sanctuary here at Rowdy Girl. We honor them, not as a meal, but as living, breathing beings who now get to live out their natural lives in peace as ambassadors of the millions of turkeys that are never seen on this day.

Every year, we serve them a feast of pureed pumpkin, cranberries, blueberries, and grapes. It's our ritual now—a celebration of life, not loss. And every year, I feel the weight of the irony: that on a day meant to celebrate gratitude, most people are giving thanks over the carved-up remains of someone who wanted to live.

That thought wrecks me. Because for every Chi Chi, Alana, and Cooper, there are millions more who never get the chance to simply *be*. Their bodies are broken into pieces before they ever know safety, affection, or freedom. *ThanksLiving* is my way of reclaiming that narrative—of saying: I see you. I honor you.

I will never again confuse violence with gratitude.

*ThanksLiving* means to me: being truly grateful for life—not for bodies broken by tradition.

Every year now, I look forward to this moment of *ThanksLiving*—where compassion takes center stage, and life—*not loss*—is what we gather around.

Eventually, I learned to create an entire vegan holiday spread and Tommy's family learned to make room at the table for a few extra dishes. Instead of hanging out over a dead turkey with the family, I choose my fellowship opportunities with them carefully. I make sure that there is plenty of plant-based food that mimics what everyone else is eating. When they make the big production over the bird and start carving into the roasted flesh, I cringe and walk away. I say a prayer and thank God I am vegan and now have eyes to see the truth.

I also had to learn to let our family continue with their traditions and live with their choices. The first Thanksgiving after Tommy became vegan was a total disaster. We have pictures of us all smiling as a family but it was awkward. We were making everybody feel bad about the turkey. (OK, *I* was making everybody feel bad because Tommy never wanted to make any waves). Even now, I must remember that I'm there to be with my family, not convert anyone to veganism. As long as they don't ask me questions or say some snide remark, I can be a conscious family member. If, on the other hand, someone steps over the line and tries to one-up me with some off-color anti-vegan comment, all bets are off, and I will shut them down in a heartbeat so we can go back to having the focus on the family instead of arguing.

It's not the family's fault. We've all been conditioned to believe that we must follow our ancestor's traditions year after year. We are hardened to the death of these sentient animals. Every November, we go into the grocery store and are bombarded with hundreds of dead bird bodies. The only thing that shocks us is the price!

I'm grateful we've created new traditions. At our *ThanksLiving* celebration, we center the lives of the animals who call our sanctuary home. But when we visit my family, it's a different story. They still eat animals—but Tommy and I show up with a vibrant vegan feast of our own. And you know what? Even our families dig in. They'll eat the compassionate food we bring, and sometimes they even ask for seconds.

I don't shrink myself or stay quiet. I show up bold, rooted, and unapologetically vegan. It's not about starting arguments—it's about holding steady in the truth.

And sometimes, just being fully yourself in a room that doesn't reflect your values is the loudest kind of activism there is.

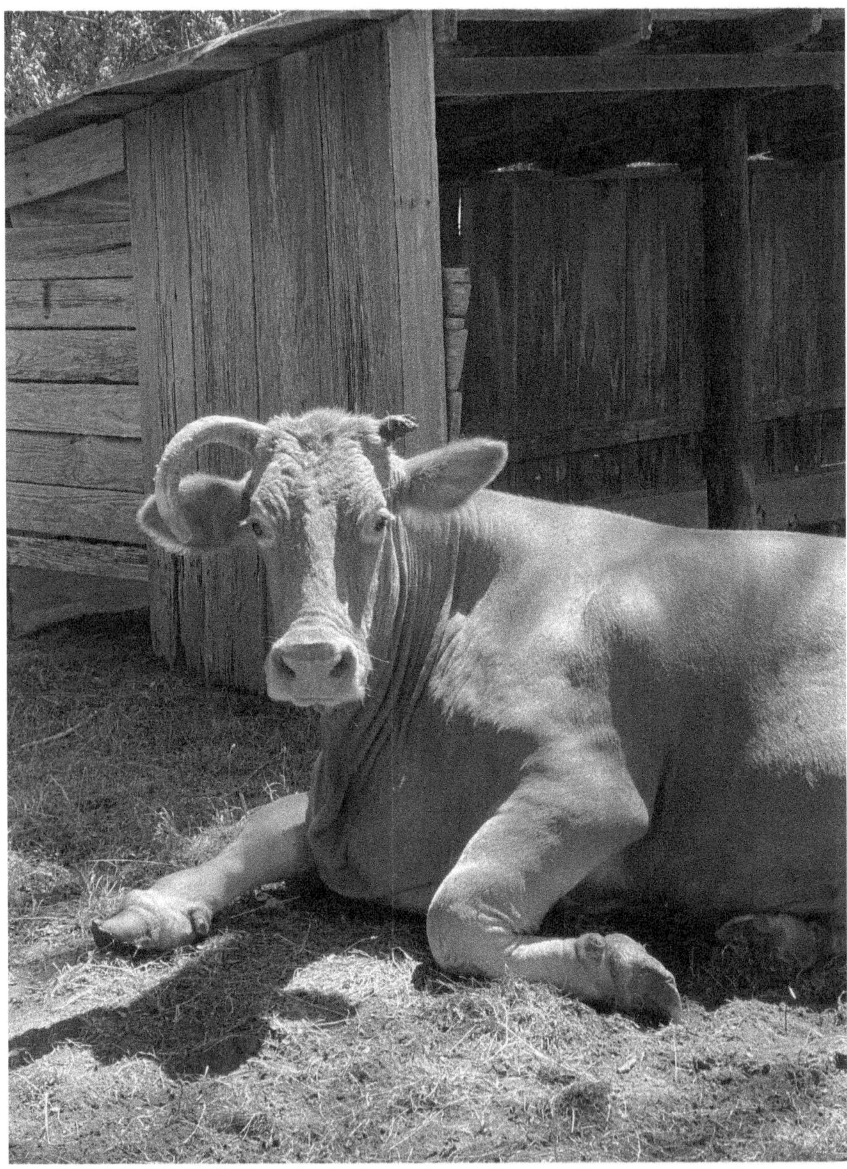

**Figure 12 Sophie.** *Purportedly 43 years old, a living testament to endurance and grace. Her presence stirred my God spot and reminded me that cows can be seen as mythical elders, not commodities.*

# 30

# *How 18,000 Cows Triggered My God Spot*

*There is nothing like the feeling of a cow's body on yours, absolutely nothing! They absorb all suffering!*

*February 19, 2015*

On April 10, 2023, 18,000 dairy cows went up in flames when the South Fork Dairy Farm in Dimmit, Texas, exploded because of malfunctioning methane equipment. Dimmit is near Laredo and the border of Piedras Negras, Mexico, with a population of 4,167 people. There were more cows in that one building than people in the entire town. (Sidenote: this is where my daddy was born).

The insanity of that stark fact is unbelievable. The state fire marshal believes the fire was started by methane ignited from overheating electrical equipment.

Investigators said that the machine, called a "honey badger," is a "vacuum that sucks the manure and urine out." Can you imagine sucking the manure and urine from 18,000 cows? What the actual fuck?! How in the heck does anyone in their right mind think it's normal to mess around with that much poop and pee from all those cows and try to manage it all? For what? Milk?

Do you know what is really disgusting? According to an article by Visual Capitalist on October 2, 2022, "The U.S. had 1.5 billion pounds of cheese in cold storage across the country. That's around $3.4 billion worth of cheese."[1]

While milk consumption declines, stockpiles of cheese go up because they don't have any other way to conserve the excess milk.

According to Visual Capitalist, "Over the last thirty years, milk production in the U.S. has increased by fifty percent."

Please note that this is milk production, *not* consumption. They continue,

"Yet, while milk production has climbed, milk consumption has declined." Furthermore, they state, "In response to this predicament, the U.S. government and dairy companies have been purchasing the extra milk and storing it as cheese for years. Today, the U.S. cheese stockpile weighs more than the Eiffel Tower, Statue of Liberty, Tower of Pisa, and the Great Sphinx of Giza combined!"

Imagine 1.5 *billion* pounds of cheese stockpiled in America while dairy cows go up in smoke, and we deprive baby calves of their mothers' milk all over the world. The reality of this equation shakes me to my core.

Nearly 6.5 million farm animals have died in fires since 2013. That's outrageous. Why in the world are we putting animals in situations where they are literally a time bomb just waiting to explode? Cows in food production are purported to emit 150 billion gallons of methane per day.[2]

Methane levels in the atmosphere are now more than two and a half times their preindustrial level. Consider the fact that 37 percent of methane emissions from human activity are the direct result of our livestock and agricultural practices (source: Environmental Protection Agency).[3]

When I heard about the 18,000 cows burning alive, I was distraught and on edge for days. I was unable to think straight while doing my job. As an empath, I can't even tell you how horrifying it is to feel the anguish of not only the cows' pain perishing in such an unbelievably painful way and it isn't just how, it's why—human greed and apathy. It sickens me to the place where my soul lives. *Who the hell are we?*

Humans have become like robots that don't care about animals' lives unless they produce a product, be it milk, shoes, furniture, entertainment, steak, or experiments. You name it. Humans will find a way to exploit, use, and abuse animals.

Before I went vegan, I wouldn't have batted an eye at these stats—methane emissions, consumption rates, animal casualties in barn fires—they would've seemed like just numbers. But now? I can't unsee the truth behind them. I'm obsessed. Every data point is a glimpse into the massive, systemic violence we've normalized. And before I could even write this section, I had to take a moment to breathe—because the scale of the collateral damage is *that overwhelming.*

So, I called my partner Connie Spence, founder of the Agriculture Fairness Alliance, a 501c4 vegan-backed lobbying group.

Connie told me that methane digesters have been causing fires since 2011. She informed me that these new "renewable" energy companies are selling contracts for exclusive energy use to transportation companies like city buses, delivery vehicles, transit stations, etc. Then, on the other side, they are going around the United States to find mega dairy farms and selling them the idea that they can all make a lot of money by simply collecting the manure and placing these million-dollar digesters right next to the cows. They are contracting with cities to buy the energy from cow shit.

Now they are selling cow shit like salvation—spun as a holy mission while animals suffer. The audacity of it all blows my mind. So, if you are a vegan and trying to live a vegan lifestyle, you could be contributing to the dairy industry and not even know it because they're using cows to create so-called "clean energy."

Yep. These money-grabbing companies are presenting these opportunities to dairy farms, and as a result, these "renewable" energy companies are forcing vegans to redefine how we operate in society. It's one thing to ask for oat milk at your favorite coffee shop. However, who knew that we live in a society where we have to ask if our transportation and delivery services are vegan too? Everything we do functions off the backs, skins, bones, flesh, blood, organs, and excretions of animals.

These explosive time bombs are waiting for the right moment to blow up another 18,000 cows. Who cares? Another bailout is sure to take care of losses and get farmers back in business in no time. As shown in the figure, according to the Agricultural Fairness Alliance, the town of Dimmit, Texas, received over *$35.18 million* of tax-payer-funded government money from 2019 to 2022.[4]

It sounds like the egregious amount of fraud and negligence in the livestock and animal feed industry has a neon light shining on their charade.

How insane is it to use the oversupply of methane to create "clean energy" and stockpile cheese because there's too much milk production and not enough people drinking it?

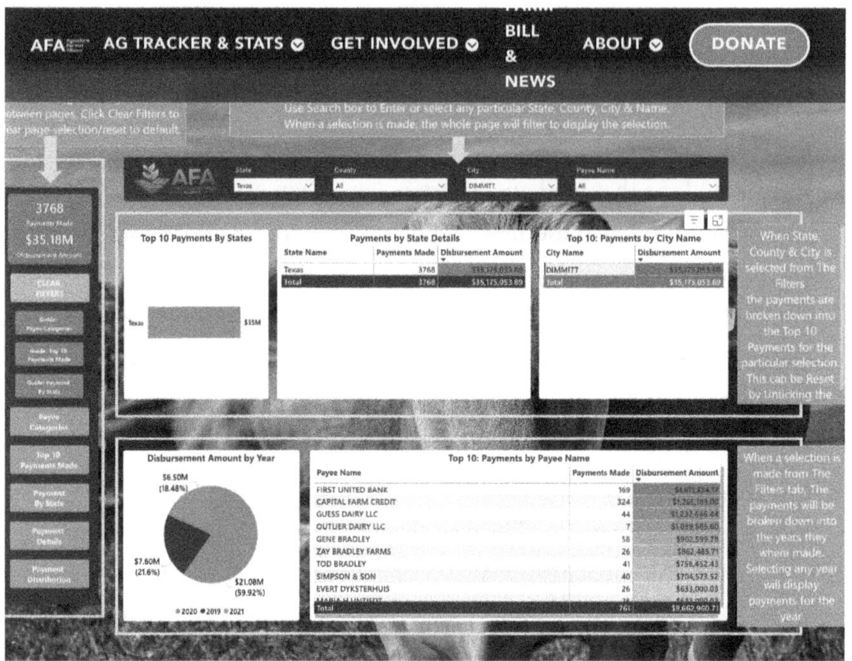


"Sounds like psychosis to me!" said Connie. I quote, "The ongoing psychosis of us trying to figure out how to use animals will never end until we stop using animals."

We cannot continue to use, abuse, and rape sentience for profit and pleasure. It feels like we are eating ourselves alive and expecting to go to heaven doing it.

Ancient Greek mathematician and philosopher, Pythagoras, who lived in 490 BC, taught that all animals, not just humans, had souls, which were immortal and reincarnated after death. He theorized that since a human might become an animal at death, and an animal might become a human, he believed that killing and eating nonhuman animals defiled the soul and prevented union with a higher form of reality. Basically, he was saying that to eat a cow is to, in effect, eat ourselves. As long as we eat animals, we create a cyclical hell on Earth and will never reach the next realm until we return to the original Eden.

Jesus, my precious Lord, would be doing a whole lot more than flipping some tables over in a flea market if He had been near the South Fork Dairy Farm that night of the explosion. WWJD (what would Jesus do), people? Jesus, who was born in a manger with cows and other farm animals all around Him, was a friend to them.

I was steeped in an Evangelical Christian Conservative community. It wasn't just about church on Sundays—it was our way of life. We believed the Bible to be the Word of God, that salvation came only through Jesus, and that it was our duty to bring others into the fold. We were taught exactly what to believe, how to act, and what our place was—especially if you were a woman. Girls like me were raised to be submissive to male authority, not speak unless spoken to and to never question the men who claimed to speak for God. We were expected to serve, not lead. Feel, but not think too much. Follow authority and not get out of bounds.

Growing up in that conservative Christian community, I never considered myself political. I'm not convinced that voting makes a difference one way or the other. However, I do it anyway because it's a right I have, and I exercise it. Honestly, I don't know if the left or the right is really that far apart in the animal agriculture world. They are all in bed with the same beast.

Dismayed after South Fork Dairy, I turned to scripture as I often do when the world is falling apart.

I opened my Bible to the book of Genesis.

> And God blessed them, and God said unto them, "Be fruitful, and multiply, and replenish the earth, and subdue it: and have dominion over the fish of the sea, and over the fowl of the air, and over every living thing that moveth upon the earth." And God said, "Behold, I have given you every herb bearing seed, which is upon the face of all the earth, and every tree, in which is the fruit of a tree yielding seed; to you it shall be for *meat*. And to every beast of the earth, and to every fowl of the air, and to everything that creepeth upon the earth, wherein there is life, I have given every green herb for *meat*": and it was so.
>
> (Genesis 1:28–30 KJV)

This is the true intention of God for man and animals.

We are not here to figure out how to get bailouts when our cows burn up from fires, drown in floods, or freeze to death. We are here to be good stewards, not to dominate but to be like their Lord.

As I sat with my Bible and reflected on the devastating loss of so many cows in Dimmit, my heart ached. I couldn't help but think of every single life lost—innocent beings who felt fear, heat, and pain. And yet, the same God who cares about every eyelash and hair on our heads surely cared about them too.

In the late hours of the night, when everything was winding down on the Sanctuary, I'd open my Bible and try to make sense of it all. But how can you make sense of this kind of suffering? Why aren't other people who love God upset by this kind of destruction too? I couldn't get the image of these cows screaming and in pain out of my mind.

"God, how can this be? How can so many lives go up in smoke in silence? No one there to mourn the loss? My heart can't carry this alone, Lord," I'd call out to Him. "Help me understand how to care for your planet and all of the creatures."

I begged the Lord to break our hearts for His creation, so we could return to His original intention for us.

"Lord, these are your creations. You must be grieving too. That's not why you made them. Please forgive us, we know not what we do. Please awaken us from this deep dark sleep."

Then I felt the Lord respond to me through the scripture—we are made in the image of God—not to dominate or destroy—but to reflect divine love, compassion, and stewardship. Our Creator did not intend for this kind of suffering for His creatures.

God gave us an abundance of food that springs forth from the earth—plants that He lovingly called "meat" in Genesis. I believe with all my heart that He never intended flesh and blood to be our nourishment.

In my grief, I returned to the teachings of Jesus—the heart of mercy, the call to love all of creation. I believe that when we align with that spirit, we find a way of living that honors both God and every living soul He made.

I used that grief as fuel, and spoke up on behalf of the 18,000.

On April 14, 2023, I wrote this on our Facebook page to share with our community and beyond:

> "I am devastated by the loss of life in Dimmit, Texas, and the unforgivable inaction to save any of the cows who perished in this unprecedented and catastrophic fire; 18,000 living, breathing mothers were treated as objects

to be disposed of, and business as usual continues. When there is any sort of disaster in the animal ag industries, here comes big government handing out more dollars to cover the damage of this deeply unsustainable industry. Do you want to know how much taxpayer funded government money Dimmit, Texas, alone has received between 2019 and 2022? You can find out via the US Agriculture Payments Tracker on the Agriculture Fairness Alliance website. Here's the grand total for those three years: $35.18 million dollars. Let that number sink in a minute.

I am furious when I think about all the destruction of life by the animal agriculture industry funded by government lobbying. When will we as a society evolve to a point where we view life as precious and not as a commodity? When will we recognize the inherent right of all beings to live free of exploitation? When will we stop funding Big Ag? We've got to rise up! Enough is enough! Wake up Texas, Wake Up World!"

May the lives lost in Dimmit, Texas, not be forgotten.

*But ask the animals, and they will teach you; the birds of the air, and they will tell you.*

*(Job 12:7 KJV)*

# 31

# *The Birth of RAP: My Vision for the Future*

*A couple of months ago, I launched the Rancher Advocacy Program where we are helping other ranchers go from animal cruelty models, known as ranching, to other sustainable models that will heal the planet and save the animals. There's lots of work to be done, and I need all of you to continue to support our work.*

*September 9, 2018*

In July of 2018, we officially started the Rancher Advocacy Program. RAP's mission is to inspire and educate farmers and ranchers, not alienate them. We recognize that both the animals and the ranchers are stuck in an archaic system without much choice. The government's indoctrination runs deep. Ranchers are rewarded by and often dependent on subsidies.

In places like Brazoria County, Texas, it's downright suffocating. Out there, ranchers don't just raise cattle by themselves—the cattle are raised by the system itself. We saw it with our own eyes. When floods came, when droughts hit, when markets crashed—ranchers around us got bailed out. Paid per head. Covered for feed losses. Compensated for dead calves.[1]

Programs like the USDA's Livestock Forage Disaster Program and Livestock Indemnity Program are designed to keep ranchers in the game—not help them get out. From 1995 to 2023, over $1.3 million was handed out to ranchers in Brazoria County through just one program—the Non-Insured Crop Disaster Assistance Program (NAP).[2] Big cattle operations in Alvin, Angleton, and

Freeport cashed those checks while the rest of us struggled to stay afloat or break free.[3]

And here's the kicker: there's zero government support for ranchers who want to do the right thing. No help if you want to stop breeding animals. No aid if you choose life over livestock. If you want to let your land heal and your heart wake up? You're on your own.

That's how the system is rigged. It rewards conformity. It punishes compassion. It bankrolls exploitation with taxpayer money—while starving out anyone who dares to walk away. Ranchers aren't evil—they're trapped. Just like I was.

In many ways, the cattle ranchers and other animal farmers are being farmed themselves by Big Ag. They have to produce food using animals for profit, or they fail. They're forced to turn animals into profit or go broke—those are the rules—and as I've stated before, the rules are rigged in favor of Big Ag not the farmer. This isn't food production; it's a blood-stained business model disguised as tradition. Survival at the expense of innocent lives is a moral collapse we've normalized for too long.

I broke the chain. I walked away. And now I'm telling the truth about how deep the lie goes. It's time to bring this buried controversy to the surface.

We had to do something dramatically different.

Tommy and I are the first cattle ranch in documented history to transition our cow/calf operation from animal farming to a nonprofit vegan farm sanctuary.

(I had no idea this would be our destiny when I went vegan).

Additionally, we have begun growing food in our Rowdy Girl Veganic Farm and educating the public. Tommy is committed to creating a veganic garden that will eventually supply our local community with fresh produce and educate local business owners on the value of growing food veganically.

Who knew that we would *also* pioneer what is now the "farm transition movement"?

Transitioning from a Big Ag mindset to kinder, more sustainable models is no easy feat. Most days, I can't believe we managed it. As you can see, we were able to transition out of animal farming and into a different way of sustaining ourselves. Along the way, I've realized that many ranchers and animal farmers don't necessarily have the background or resources to navigate nonprofit fundraising—it's a whole different world.

As a former rancher, I see things through a different lens from that of the typical vegan. I have compassion for families whose identities and livelihoods are wrapped up in this system. Hell, the whole Texas persona is wrapped up in beef, barbecue, rodeos, cook-offs and the like—When Texas goes vegan, the rest of the nation will follow. And y'all, it *is* happening!

Ranchers are not bad people, far from it. We're raised on animal agriculture. We become dependent on government subsidies. We know how to ranch and many of us don't know much else. Tommy and I have a unique chemistry and a novel story that made fundraising a viable path for us. I had years of experience performing and starting and running small businesses. But for most people, that simply isn't the case. Even with our advantages, we've had a lot of help along the way. We understand the position ranchers are in, stuck between animal agriculture and the world of animal rights and earnestly, we want to help.

When our story went viral, it hit a compassionate nerve previously not easily triggered in the world of cowboys, cattle ranches, and Texan culture. I received hundreds of messages, emails, and calls from ranchers, their wives, and their family and friends, reaching out to me for support and guidance.

We officially launched the Rancher Advocacy Program (RAP) on a standalone website in July 2018 but the idea came to me years before. Back in 2015, when Rowdy Girl Sanctuary was just a few months old, I had a booth at Marshall Healthfest in Marshall, Texas, to get the word out about what we were doing. Well-known, plant-based celebrities had traveled from across the country to discuss the benefits of a plant-based diet, and I hoped our story might connect with someone who could help.

Our story was all the buzz at the festival, and I met quite a few leaders I admired: Miyoko, Chef A.J., Rich Roll, T. Colin Campbell, and Gene Baur. Our booth was next to Kat Mendenhall, the vegan boot maker who used to call her company Kick Butt Boots. Before meeting Kat, I didn't know if I would ever again enjoy the luxury of owning different styles of cowgirl boots. I can honestly say that being a vegan cowgirl has never been easier, and I have Kat to thank for that.

Within a couple of hours of opening, a tall, thin Texas cowboy walked up to me with a toothpick hanging out the side of his mouth. He wore a straw

Stetson hat, leather cowboy boots with silver tips, freshly ironed polyester wranglers, a starched cowboy shirt with snaps all the way down and big Texas cufflinks. He finished off his attire with a fancy Western jacket. Nobody looked less like a vegan.

This man was walking the walk of a long, tall Texan. Evidently, his wife had perused our booth about an hour before, discovered that we used to be a cattle ranch and were now vegan, and she sent him over to talk to me.

"I hear you used to be a cattle ranch and that you don't sell your cows anymore. What are you doing with 'em?" he asked.

"Well, I saved 'em all. I started a fundraiser, and when it was funded, I bought my husband's small herd and started a nonprofit farm animal sanctuary," I replied.

"So, what do you do with the cows now?"

"We love them like they're our family," I beamed. "They each have a name and a medical file, and they are saved from slaughter forever."

He wiggled his eyebrows as if to express disbelief and began to tell me of his dilemma.

"We are an eighth-generation cattle ranch," he proudly stated, "and our kids don't want to inherit the farm because they're now vegetarian, with some considering a vegan diet. What do you recommend I do with my land?" he snapped. "Do you have any answers for me?"

I looked at him dumbfounded and said, "Wow, your kids don't want to inherit the cruelty. Do you think they would want to inherit the farm if you could do something different besides raising cows for food?"

He was ticked off, which was fair. He struck a nerve with me too. He looked at me with narrow eyes and said, "Listen here, this land has been in my family for eight generations. It's all we know. What else are we gonna do on six hundred acres? Do you have any ideas or solutions for me?"

I didn't have a solution. All I could think of was that he could start a 501c3 nonprofit farm animal sanctuary. But not every rancher or animal farmer has the expertise and life experience to fundraise, promote, and be a public figure to help their cause. Our solution wasn't the solution for everyone.

I was speechless for a moment. Then I said to the cowboy, "I will figure it out. There's gotta be a way for good folks like you that want to transition from animal farming into some other kind of agriculture for human consumption."

"Well, when you figure it out, let me know because I got a real problem on my hands." He sighed and walked off with a wink.

I never got that man's phone number or address.

My mind was racing. We were only a few months old as a nonprofit, and I was faced with the toughest question that our animal rights movement had faced. I became infatuated with figuring out how to give ranchers and animal farmers options on their farms, so they could leave behind a legacy of compassion and reverence for life, land, and family instead of cruelty and unsustainable farming practices.

I started delving into the unchartered waters of farm transition. The deeper I went, the more desperate I became. The more media attention Rowdy Girl got, the more questions ranchers had about transition.

Once, I was out in the pasture feeding the cows, and I got a call from the daughter of a cattle rancher who said, "I'm so glad you answered the phone. I can't believe you answered." This woman was weeping on the other end, and I could hardly make sense of her words. I slowed her down by telling her to breathe and that I wasn't going anywhere.

With all the calmness this lady could muster, she blurted out that her dad didn't know she was calling.

> I've told my daddy that I don't like sending the babies to sale, but he always tells me that this is what we do and that I need to grow up. He tells me that God put them on this Earth to be food. However, even though I'm a God-fearin' woman, something inside of me knows that them babies are the pride and joy of their mommas, just like my babies are to me, she cried.

She continued,

> I've watched 'em. The mommas love them babies. When they are loaded up to go to the sale barn, the mommas cry for days. It breaks my heart, and I can't stand it. I've told my daddy this over and over again, but he's a hard-core rancher and a good man. Hearing you on TV gave me hope. It was like

there was someone that understood my heart. I wasn't alone. Thank you for answering the phone.

I told her she wasn't alone and that she could call me anytime. The nagging question of how farmers and ranchers would make money on their land without breeding and commodifying animals loomed. It was one thing to be a sympathetic ear, but what good was that if there was no solution to the animal farming problem?

The calls continued. I received another call from a friend down the road.

"Renée," she said, "I have a friend married to a cattle rancher. She has fallen in love with these two steers and doesn't want them to be sold for slaughter. Can you buy them?" She sounded desperate.

"Who is this person?" I asked. She told me that her friend wanted to remain anonymous.

I told her I wasn't in the business of buying other people's livestock, but that I'd talk to her friend.

She started to sniffle. "I don't think that she will talk to you." Her voice was quivering now, and she was trying to hold it together.

I asked her, "Is that cattle rancher's wife, you?"

She cried as if a dam had been let loose in her heart. I felt every tear and every sob. I cried with her.

After a few moments, I said, "You know I can't buy your steers. If I buy those two, what about the rest of the herd? Aren't they just as special?"

"I've gotten attached to these two," she reminisced. "If I could just save them, at least it would give me somewhat of a clear conscience around what we are doing," she said with hope.

"I can't do it," I explained. "Why don't you tell your husband how you feel?"

She became nervous.

"Renée, promise me you will not tell my husband that I called you. In fact, I should've never called. Forget I called you about this. What was I thinking? Promise me, promise me," she pleaded.

"I promise. You have my word," I said.

I saw this lady at her place of business a couple of weeks later and we acted like nothing had happened. We smiled and exchanged "howdy do's," but her phone call genuinely impacted me. She was a prominent neighbor and businesswoman. There was so much shame wrapped up in her love for those animals. It broke my heart.

In those days, I did a lot of listening, but it was Cindy's call that finally made me take action. Her husband, a sixth-generation cattle rancher named Richard, was about to send a cow named Honey to the sale barn because she had a bad hip, and they could not breed her anymore.

On the phone, Cindy's cries were palpable. For about thirty minutes, she wept in a state of utter torment. Honey had awakened Cindy as Rowdy Girl had awakened me. Her husband was going to haul her beloved cow to the slaughterhouse.

She told me that she had tried many other well-known sanctuaries in the country and that no one would help her. She felt helpless and without options. I told her we were at capacity and couldn't take Honey, but I would do what I could to help her find a solution. I asked her if Richard would be amicable. She assured me he would. I set out to solve her problem.

I knew a cattle ranch that had gone vegan shortly after us in central Texas. This couple had inherited the ranch from the husband's father and they were charged with figuring out how to make a business out of it. Neither wanted to send the remaining cows to slaughter, so I was trying to figure out how to help them. Even though I was never able to help them find another way to make money, I did make a vital connection between them and Cindy.

I told them that the clock was ticking for sweet Honey and they both agreed to become Honey's new caretakers. Tommy, Ryuji (an intern at the time and budding filmmaker), and I headed off to Huntsville to meet the ranchers and help Honey.

When we got there, it was cold and drizzly. Cindy and Richard greeted us outside. Cindy hugged me with tears in her eyes and was so grateful. Richard was the opposite. He looked us up and down, and I could tell he didn't trust us one bit. After about thirty minutes of conversation outside and meeting Honey, we were invited inside to have coffee and get better acquainted. All the while, Ryuji was filming and documenting.

Once we got inside, Richard said he told his wife what he was *really* thinking—that we would probably be picking up Honey to take her to a sale barn. He couldn't fathom the thought of a vegan rancher. He thought it all sounded too good to be true and was relieved to meet us and discover we were sincere.

After talking to Tommy and me, he warmed up and began to speak openly and frankly about his thoughts on the environment, his personal struggles, and politics. He was glad that Honey had a place to go. He also said that Honey had a daughter named Ginger and that she could go too if the folks in central Texas were receptive. Cindy beamed, and tears fell. Together, we rounded up the two cows and trailered them off to the sanctuary.

After Honey and Ginger left, Richard and Cindy faced many challenges before finally ending their cattle ranch operation altogether. Rowdy Girl became home for the last of their livestock. Missy, Cinnie, Sammie, Minnie, and Monty found refuge and peace at Rowdy Girl. Cinnie gave birth to baby Nutmeg nine months after she got here. None of them will ever be in the ring to be sold as chattel. They will forever be seen as sentient beings and part of our RAP history and legacy.

The conversation with Richard and Cindy changed me. I saw it was not only possible but vital to bridge the gap between their community and mine. I became determined to do more than help people place cows. People had been asking me what "our main program" at the nonprofit would be, and the need for RAP was clear. I wanted to find a viable solution for farms to keep their doors open.

As I took more and more calls from ranchers looking for a way out, it became clear: they needed options that would let them stay rooted on their land—options they could be proud of. I started exploring what those alternatives could be. Not theories—real possibilities. Paths that could shift the paradigm while honoring the legacy of the land. These are some of our strategic plans that emerged:

## Plant-Based Farm—Distribution Contract with a Plant-Based Food Company

In the very early days of Rowdy Girl, one of the visions that came to me was simple but radical: What if farmers could partner directly with plant-based food companies? What if the same land used to raise animals for slaughter could be used to grow the future—and do it under contract, with real economic support?

The idea of *plant-based food distribution contracts* between farmers and plant-based brands isn't just a novel idea—it's a game-changer. It bridges the gap between supply and demand, between mission and livelihood. It gives farmers a way out that isn't just theoretical or idealistic—it's *viable.* It gives them a customer, a purpose, and a paycheck that doesn't depend on suffering.

Right now, most farmers are locked into Big Ag contracts that guarantee one thing: exploitation. But imagine replacing that with contracts that support the production of legumes, grains, mushrooms, fruits, and vegetables—all the foods driving the plant-based movement forward. Imagine food companies investing in the soil, not the slaughterhouse. That's how we create a just transition.

This vision gives power back to the farmer. It lets them keep their land. It lets them keep their pride. And it puts them on the right side of history—feeding the world without destroying it.

We created countless spreadsheets and documents full of research that our volunteers put together about local farms that we could potentially partner with one day. Our aim was to create a plant-based food alliance as big as animal ag and that dream is still alive in me!

## Solar and Wind Farms

At our yearly RAP summits, we'd discuss our plans and invite speakers from around the world to inspire us to think differently about what is possible regarding farm transition and the plant-based food movement.

During that time, I saw solar and wind farms as real paths forward so that farmers could stay on their land and make money. These options used the land for good, producing clean energy instead of producing animals for slaughter. But like every solution, these came with drawbacks.

Solar and wind farms require large upfront investments and often attract corporate interests that can edge out small farmers, leasing the land without investing in the people or the communities. They can also take land out of food production entirely, turning once-cultivated soil into energy fields. And while they reduce emissions, they don't inherently address food justice, animal liberation, or community health unless they're rooted in an ethical framework.

Still, they cracked open the door to a new kind of land use—a step away from slaughter and a step toward sustainability. And that mattered to me.

## Veganic Agriculture

Another innovation we sought to implement was Veganic Agriculture to teach farmers how to grow food without using animal inputs.

If you live near chicken farms, like I do, there are some days you can't even walk outside because there's such a gagging and burning smell of chicken manure used to fertilize the hay pastures around us. Veganic soil on the other hand, is built from the Earth itself—composted produce vegetation, twigs, leaves, no animal waste, no blood, no bone, just plants feeding plants the way nature intended.

It was Kip Andersen who first got us thinking hard about veganic farming—not as some fringe idea, but as a powerful way to prove that you could grow food without animal inputs. Since then, Tommy's planted multiple veganic gardens on our sanctuary land, and they get better and better each time. Every single one has proven: you don't need animal by-products to grow food—you just need commitment, good soil, and a willingness to work the land every day.

Sometimes I picture myself in my overalls with my guitar, standing by the side of the road with a little farm stand that says: *Rowdy Girl Veganic Farm.* I'll be selling fresh produce straight from the sanctuary—food grown without blood, bone, or cruelty. Just Texas sunshine, rich black soil, and lots of Rowdy love.

And next to the tomatoes and greens? A simple flyer. Not confrontational. Not pushy. Just a kind invitation to think differently about the food you grow and the animals you raise.

It would gently explain what a veganic farm really is—how we grow fruits and vegetables using compost from plant matter. It would share what it means to live the sanctuary life. A place where animals that are rescued from slaughter, now roam free.

## Rewilding the Land

Rewilding is about giving the land back to nature. Before rewilding, ranch land is stripped of its natural biodiversity. Monoculture feed crops replace wild grasses. The animals who once lived freely are driven out. The land becomes silent, controlled, and exhausted. But rewilding brings it back to life.

I saw it with my own eyes when Dr. Sailesh Rao took me, Jane Velez-Mitchell, and a small group of activists to a once-ravaged cattle ranch in Costa Rica. What we walked into was nothing short of sacred—vibrant forest where there was once grazing land, howler monkeys calling from the canopy, and native plants reclaiming the soil. The fences were gone, the balance was returning, and the Earth was breathing again.

That experience changed me. Rewilding isn't just ecological restoration—it's a living testimony that healing is possible. It's not about controlling the land—it's about getting out of the way and letting nature remember who she is. And that, to me, is the heart of sanctuary.

When you get out of the way, and let nature take over, it's better than anything that we could ever do.

## Real and Rowdy Feed Stores

I have this dream that one day, in every rural town across America, the local feed store—the hub where farmers gather, talk weather, buy supplies—will look completely different. Not because we've erased the culture, but because we've reclaimed it.

Imagine a feed store not owned by industrial ag interests, but by plant-based farmers—people growing real food for the future and in rural communities. Walk through the doors and instead of being hit with the smell of leather and barrels of dried pig ears sold as dog treats, you see something else: shelves lined with ethically sourced, pesticide-free feed made by conscious growers.

Feed created for animals who are living out their lives in sanctuaries—not fattened for slaughter.

And on the walls? Screens playing documentaries about the local plant-based farmers who are reclaiming the land, restoring the soil, and feeding their communities without harm. Flyers advertising workshops on veganic growing, clean composting, and rewilding your pasture. A bulletin board showcasing sanctuary stories, not sale barn prices.

These stores wouldn't just sell supplies—they'd nurture a new narrative. A space where compassion and agriculture finally meet. A place where people still gather—but to talk about soil health, animal well-being, and a future where rural economies thrive without blood on their hands.

It's not just a feed store. It's a seedbed for change.

## Community Farmers Market

Now we're taking it a step further. From the pulse of the local feed store, a Community Farmers Market begins to rise—not just as a place to buy produce, but as a living, breathing extension of the movement.

It starts with conscious growers—plant-based farmers who've reclaimed the soil, who know their land and their crops like kin. Their feed store becomes the epicenter: a gathering place, a teaching space, and now, a launchpad for local food economies that don't depend on Big Ag or big box stores.

And this isn't just about helping rural communities thrive—it's about transforming cities too. For too long, urban neighborhoods—especially underserved ones—have become dumping grounds for processed junk and fast food chains, creating public health disasters masked as convenience. But what if we flipped the script?

What if, instead of drive-throughs and dollar menus built on suffering, we created fast food produce stands—grab-and-go hubs for fresh fruits, veggies, and handmade, plant-based meals? Food that actually feeds. Food that heals. Grown by rural farmers who are part of the same movement, delivered directly into urban food deserts that were never meant to be starved in the first place.

This model reconnects the land with the people. It turns farmers into leaders. It turns feed stores into cultural centers. It turns cities into allies in the fight for real food. We don't have to settle for corporate crumbs. We can take back our power—and that power starts with our hands in the dirt and our roots in justice.

## Lab-Grown Meat Facility

Imagine this: a 1,000-acre cattle ranch in the heart of Texas—once fully entrenched in the business of breeding, branding, and sending animals to slaughter. But instead of doubling down on a dying system, this ranch chooses a different path. They save part of their herd, give them sanctuary, and on the very land where animals once waited to die, they build something revolutionary: a lab-grown meat facility. Not hidden. Not shameful. But celebrated.

Visitors can tour the sanctuary, look a cow in the eye, and know she'll never be killed. Then they walk next door, where meat is being grown in a lab—not from suffering, but from science. They sit down to enjoy a burger that tastes just like beef because it *is* beef—only no one had to die for it. It's food with a conscience, and it turns the ranch into a tourist destination, a model for the future.

And yet—just as this kind of vision is becoming real—Texas lawmakers are trying to shut it down. Senate Bill 261 aims to ban the sale and production of cultured meat in Texas. Not because it's unsafe—it's already been approved by the FDA and USDA. But because it threatens the very system that profits from pain. It threatens the illusion that there is no other way.

This bill isn't about protecting consumers. It's about protecting Big Ag's chokehold on our land, our food, and our future. But here's the truth: you can't legislate innovation out of existence. You can't stop people from dreaming of a better way. The land itself is ready. The science is here. And the public is waking up. So it's time for Texas to go vegan!

What if the very heart of cattle country became the place where animals were no longer killed for burgers but honored—and where the next generation came to learn, eat, and believe that a different future *is not only possible—it's already growing*?

As an ethical vegan, I would never eat it myself, but this isn't about me. It's about shifting the entire system. If we're going to change the world, we have to meet people where they are. For the billions who aren't ready to give up meat, cell-based meat is a lifeline—a way out of slaughter without sacrificing taste or tradition. And it's not just for people—it's a game-changer for pet food, too. No more grinding up baby chicks or factory-farmed scraps to feed our dogs and cats. Cultured meat offers an ethical alternative across the board. It's not perfection—but it's progress.

And sometimes, that's how revolutions begin.

## Transition Ain't Easy

In 2018, we met a family from Arkansas who had shut down their cattle and chicken operation and were struggling. They needed help buying hay for their cows because they were running out of money. They had gone vegan, stopped selling chickens, but they didn't know what to do next. Their reserves were running low, and they had two hundred cows to feed, bills to pay, and no income.

Tommy thought I was crazy running off and helping somebody else get hay when we needed hay ourselves but I wasn't deterred. I knew I could help them. I had one mission in mind. I decided I would start a fundraiser on the ground in Arkansas, get hay to feed the cows, and find a donor to help them with their bills so they could keep the lights on.

Within forty-eight hours, we raised about $20,000 for hay and from that day forward, we entered into what would become one of the most challenging and emotionally charged relationships in RAP's history.

In early 2019, with the help of a philanthropic funder, RAP was able to get funds to establish a research and development project at the farm. They would be our first chicken-to-mushroom transition.

The project was fraught with highs, lows, obstacles, moments of triumph, and eventually, a realization that there wasn't enough private funding to go the distance. In order for these transitions to work at scale, ranchers need government support.

Were we discouraged? Yes, but we learned a hell of a lot.

We achieved incredible progress with the initial wave of invested funds. We spent two years transforming a twenty-thousand-square-foot chicken production barn into a prototype for a large-scale exotic mushroom facility unlike any other in North America at the time. We grew thousands of pounds of exotic mushroom strains—proof that something new could take root in a place once defined by animal agriculture. It wasn't without flaws, and we faced more challenges than we could have anticipated. But for a time, we saw what was possible. That glimpse didn't solve everything, but it offered hope—real, tangible hope—that transformation can happen, even in the most unlikely of places.

Still hope alone wasn't enough to carry the vision forward.

Even with all the challenges, we arrived at a model that functioned within the scope of a specific environment. It was still fraught with human limitations we couldn't solve. So many farmers are drowning in debt, bound by contracts they didn't write, trapped in a cycle they can't escape. Big Ag doesn't offer freedom—it offers servitude. These aren't independent landowners—they're indentured servants on land their families have worked for generations. The only dreams they're allowed are the ones subsidized by blood money and controlled by corporate masters. They call it tradition. I call it entrapment.

But real freedom? That's a different story. Real freedom is still rooted in the land—but no longer shackled to suffering. It's reclaiming your birthright without selling your soul. It's farmers breaking the cycle, turning away from slaughter and toward sustainability. It's growing plants instead of pain. Harvesting energy from the sun and wind, instead of death from the backs of animals.

Real freedom is feeding your community without destroying your conscience. It's restoring your land, your health, and your spirit. It's walking off the killing floor and back into harmony—with the Earth, with yourself, and with the animals who were never ours to own.

That's the freedom I fight for. And that's the road I paved when I turned a cattle ranch into a sanctuary.

Through persistence and adaptation, a model finally took shape—one that fit the specific environment and circumstances we were working with. But no matter how sound the concept, we couldn't solve the deeper challenges. I carry hope that someone else will—someone with the vision, resources, and the unity needed to see it through.

We knew the concept had real potential—but due to funding gaps and other issues beyond our control, we ultimately had to pull the pilot. It was an incredibly difficult decision, but a necessary one.

What we needed most was support—not just from donors, but from government agencies willing to invest in meaningful change. Because the truth is, bold ideas alone aren't enough. We need infrastructure, vision, and long-term commitment to reimagine what's possible after animal agriculture. It's in all of our best interest to explore sustainable alternatives like this before more harm is done to our environment, our communities, and ourselves. My hope is that by the time you read this, someone, somewhere, is growing mushrooms on a meaningful scale using a model inspired by what we created.

When I first started RAP, no one in the world was doing anything remotely resembling farm transition. Now I know why. It's unbelievably difficult to transition farms within a government system that invests in animal agriculture as a way of life. Today, RAP's mission is to educate, inspire, and connect. We provide a place for meaningful conversations so they can understand the fundamentals of having a "wake up" call when discovering feelings about the animals they send to slaughter. Transition is a mental and moral dilemma because our entire culture is built on the backs of animals. This translates to the backs of farmers burdened with fitting into an archaic system of normalized violence.

I'm grateful that our chicken-to-mushroom farm transition sparked conversation around the world and also showed us just how necessary government support is to scale this model. *These* are the programs that need subsidizing. Everyone on the planet will benefit from farms that transition away from animal agriculture, the animals, the farmers, and humanity.

If RAP teaches us anything, it's this: We've got the nerve, the faith, and the conviction to carve out a new way—*and we're already doing it.*

Every challenge, every hard truth, every impossible conversation has shown us that deep down, we *do* care. RAP was never about fixing everything overnight—it's about cracking open the possibility that farmers can become liberators instead of laborers in a system that breaks hearts and bodies. And to any farmer out there wrestling with the weight of it all—we see you. There's a way through. We know, because we've lived it.

# 32

# *Where We've Never Been*

*Thank you, God, for my life. Thank you for giving me the eyes to see farmed animals as equals, the ears to hear their cries, and a heart that feels their pain. Thank you for the willingness to do my part in ending animal agriculture. It is important to know our why. I know mine—and it lives in the beings whose lives have been entrusted to me, who embody every reason why I will never stop advocating for their rights.*
*Love, Renée*

*August 5, 2021*

Today, our beloved matriarch, Agape, took her last breath. She was 26 years old—blind and living with advanced arthritis. We laid her to rest peacefully in the pasture she called home, in the presence of those who loved her. Her three constant companions—Ivy, Lulu, and Lotus, our potbellied pigs—remained nearby. Ivy, especially, was always close—a gentle, grounding presence around Agape in her final years.

Tommy buried her, as he always does, carrying the sacred burden of saying the final goodbye. We've laid many to rest here, but this one was different. Agape wasn't just part of the herd—she was its heart.

She came to us in 2004 from a sale barn, along with E.U., Little Red, and Notches. Branded with an "E" and notched ears, she was known then as E.D.—a number, a commodity, a symbol of everything the system deems unworthy of love. But years later, when the ranch became Rowdy Girl Sanctuary and I stepped into veganism, E.D. became someone else entirely. We renamed her Agape.

*Agape* (ἀγάπη) means unconditional, sacrificial love. In the Christian tradition, it is the highest form of love—God's love. It gives without demand, sees without conditions, and holds all life sacred. It is the love that watches over sparrows and *cows*. The love that suffers with the oppressed and lifts them into freedom. The love that liberates instead of dominates.

I named her this, so she would grow into Agape, and she did not disappoint. The name *Agape* gave her the frequency and identity she was destined for. And she lived it—beautifully, fiercely, and eloquently—all the way to the end. Naming her wasn't just a gesture. It was a reclamation. It was a restoration of her true self.

In her early years, she was known as the meanest cow in the herd. And she had every reason to be. Her babies were taken from her again and again. Every time the red trailer pulled up, Agape did everything in her power to protect them. She wasn't mean. She was a grieving mother. Once, in a burst of rage and protection, she rammed Tommy so hard he flew right out of his loafers—his shoes stayed put, and he landed hard. That was Agape: fearless in her love, unwilling to back down from injustice.

She used to look so angry with her furrowed brow, but as time went on, that anger and fear dissipated. As Agape softened, so did I. She aged so gracefully. Her blindness forced her to trust us, and her arthritis meant she had to push past pain just to get up.

Watching her, I'd learn that no matter what happens, you get up to face the day. It doesn't matter if it hurts or not. You don't complain; you do what you have to do. Stay the course. Trust what you cannot see.

Sometimes I feel like I am walking blind. Scripture reminds us in Matthew 6:33 that "Faith is the substance of things hoped for and the evidence of things not seen." Agape represented that kind of faith—she had to get to a point where she couldn't see before she softened and allowed us to draw near to her. That changed everything. Her blindness gave her the ability to see love.

Witnessing that transformation deepened my faith. Because if a badass cow like Agape could soften—could let the same hands that once stole her babies become the hands that fed her, protected her, mourned her death—then we've experienced true *agape*.

Agape, in all her strength, became the heartbeat that pulsed through this land. Her heart was always a steadying force. When she died, something in me cracked open, and what poured out wasn't despair, it was like the power of resurrection. The sacred "yes" behind every "no" I've said to this broken system. It's the quiet, unshakeable force that guides my defiance. I'm not rebelling just to rebel; I'm protecting something holy. Agape is leading me to say "no" to everything that violates love. She taught me how to soften my edges.

Rowdy Girl, on the other hand, has always been my wild side, the voice that is loud and isn't afraid to shake the walls. Rowdy Girl has always been the free spirit. But let me be clear: Rowdy Girl is also the *soul.* She is the spirit that ignited this revolution in me—a whisper at first, then a decisive call that echoes in my ears every second of every day. Rowdy Girl is ether. She's what rose up in the cracks of my old life and said: This ends with you.

Together, Rowdy Girl's mission and Agape's passing are creating the alchemy of who I am now—and who I am becoming.

It's strange that Agape's heartbeat became stronger the weaker she became physically. It's like I could feel her more. As I said goodbye to her, she left me with something—this final chapter, and a new beginning.

I used to think it was all about being rowdy—about kicking down doors, raising hell, and refusing to shut up. But as I write these final words, I realize that Agape's death and what came after wasn't just an ending. It was a revival. A resurrection of *agape* love—unconditional, unshakable, and alive in me now.

In her final hours, she gave me everything. Total vulnerability. She let me cradle her massive head, stroke her neck like a mother with her child. And I wept—not just for her, but for all the cows who never get that chance. For all the people of my species who never stop to see the sacred in a creature like her.

She transmitted something in those moments—something ancient and steady. Her heartbeat wasn't just a sound; it was a message. *Be strong. Stay grounded. And NEVER give up.*

I'm older now—softer in many ways—but more resolved than ever. Agape reminded me: strength doesn't mean hardness. It means endurance. And even our weakness, when held in love, can become a reverent kind of power.

Years before Agape passed, I already felt her life force surge through my body like a divine hand on my back saying, "Keep going." There was nothing like the fight that Agape embodied. Though fierce, her fight was always executed with the purest intent—to protect the innocent. The lessons she taught me will echo throughout my life. That fire, that love, is what I carried into every room in Washington, D.C.—because if Agape could fight for her babies with everything she had, I could fight for a world that would stop taking them.

In 2018, before Agape passed but already deeply transformed by the spirit of what she came to represent, I joined the board of the Agriculture Fairness Alliance (AFA), a 501c4 vegan-backed lobbying group determined to make vegan lobbyists a thing in D.C. *Why not?* My friend and business partner, Connie Spence, was the force that started it all and y'all, she's a force to be reckoned with! Her tenacity, brilliance, and fierce determination led the way forward in AFA and got us all collaborating with leaders on creating legislation that promoted sustainable farming instead of punishing it.

While AFA has since closed its doors, its spirit lives on in every policy we helped draft, every meeting that shook the status quo, and every advocate who now knows they do have a seat at the table. We didn't just knock—we kicked the door wide open. And the ripple effects are still moving through the system.

I was proud to be part of such a groundswell of passion dedicated to creating a new way in Washington. In 2023, we sat in Senate offices armed with language to be inserted into the 2023 Farm Bill. Connie even moved to D.C. We were perfectly poised to light a fire in D.C. because of COVID, climate change, and the avian flu pandemic that wiped out hundreds of thousands of chickens and farmer livelihoods. Politicians were starting to wake up to the fact that our agricultural system was in crisis.

We were hoping Congress would introduce language in the Farm Bill to help transition farmers to plant-based farming. But it was such a quagmire of political games. We tried to keep the faith.

And through it all—Rowdy Girl was leading me every step of the way, kicking the door open and bucking the system, while Agape's love covered me in grace and compassion.

When I stood in the halls of Congress, pleading the case for farmers, it wasn't just my voice they heard, it was the electrified focus of Rowdy Girl and the sacred weight of Agape's heartbeat.

Together, their stories lived in every talking point and every heartfelt plea. I wasn't just advocating for farmers—I was speaking for the chickens, the pigs, and the cows like Agape and Rowdy Girl. *They were behind every single word.*

If there's any hope for this government—for this world—it won't come through the same old systems, the same tired politics, or the same lobbyists who defend eight generations of tradition at the cost of truth. *It will come through you.*

The youth. The graduates. The ones standing at the edge of a choice.

We need *you* to become vegan staffers. Vegan lobbyists. Vegan politicians.

*Not later. Now.*

To move forward, we must embody both-*Rowdy Girl's defiance and Agape's unconditional love.* One disrupts the system. One heals the land, the animals, and our own hearts. Together, they transform the world.

We must live *in this world, but not be of it,* guided by a power greater than ourselves. Without them—without that fiery truth and unshakable grace, I fear the only path left is destruction. But I refuse to believe that's the only way.

I believe in something higher.

Something holy and divine.

Something possible.

That belief was born through scripture, through recovery, through Rowdy Girl, and through Agape. They taught me how to fight without hate. How to resist without losing heart. How to be rowdy for justice, and still tender for life.

So I'm charging *you* now—

Carry their spirit.

Birth in yourself a sacred defiance and a holy compassion.

Be the one who walks into broken systems with fire in your soul and love in your hands.

That's how we build the new world—one heartbeat, one charge, one reckoning, one truth at a time.

Big Ag is on shaky ground. Disease outbreaks, methane explosions, and climate extremes are putting farmers' lives and futures at risk. What once brought pride now brings fear. The current system is collapsing—and farmers know it.

Meanwhile, the plant-based movement is rising. Consumers are demanding ethical, sustainable food, and companies are racing to meet that demand. But instead of supporting American farmers to transition and supply this shift, we're still importing key ingredients—leaving willing farmers stuck in a dying system.

And it gets worse: Big Ag isn't just clinging to the past—they're waging war on the future. With massive funding and lobbying power, they're spending millions to discredit plant-based pioneers like Beyond Meat and Impossible Foods.[1] Through front groups like the Center for Consumer Freedom, they run smear campaigns that paint plant-based foods as ultra-processed "fake meat"—all while profiting off a system built on disease, deforestation, and cruelty.

They've even pushed for labeling laws to ban plant-based products from using words like "meat" or "milk," weaponizing language to confuse consumers and protect market share.[2]

But consumers aren't confused—they're evolving. And if we're serious about feeding the future, we need to empower American farmers to grow with it.

This is the time to create real distribution contracts, infrastructure, and support for farmers ready to leave animal ag behind. Not everyone can start a sanctuary—but many can grow the ingredients that power the plant-based economy.

This isn't just compassion—it's strategy. It's justice. And it's how we reclaim farming with dignity, truth, and purpose.

I say to the next generation of ranching families: You weren't born to blindly carry on what breaks your heart. You were born for *such a time as this.*

I see you—the sons and daughters standing at the edge of a tradition that shaped your whole identity, now wondering if there's another way. Maybe you've felt it: that quiet nudge in your spirit when you look an animal in the eye. That moment of stillness that makes you question what you've always been told is normal.

That's not a weakness. That's *the Holy Spirit stirring.* That's the truth trying to break through all the lies.

Tommy and I didn't become who we are overnight. We didn't have a blueprint—just a calling. Rowdy Girl Sanctuary isn't a model for everyone. Not every family will walk the same path we did. But every family has *something* they can offer: land, time, experience, testimony, faith, and their own resources.

You don't need to start a nonprofit. But you do need to start telling the truth. And that's a fact Jack!

God didn't create animals to be bought and sold. He created them to be *seen*, loved, and to reveal the innocence we've lost. If a cow like Agape could forgive the hands that once stole her babies… if a cow like Rowdy Girl can spark a revolution… if cattle ranchers like us can lay down the brand—so to speak—and pick up compassion… then *so can you.*

The Bible (Rom. 12:2) says, "Do not conform to the pattern of this world, but be transformed by the renewing of your mind."

This is your invitation. To think again. To live differently. To use what you've been given to build something *holy.*

It doesn't have to look like Rowdy Girl. But it has to look like *redemption.* Speak what's in your heart. Let go of what no longer serves life. Be the seed of a new generation—the one that sets the captives free.

And let us not forget the spirit of *Rowdy Girl*—not just a cow, but a spark that lit the fuse of change. She was bold, loud, and impossible to ignore. Her resistance cracked through generations of silence and made space for truth to rise.

Agape was different. She was stillness. Presence. The quiet power of a being who had every reason to distrust us—but chose love anyway. In her final hours, she let me see what real forgiveness looks like. Her heartbeat stays with me—it steadied my own.

Together, *Rowdy Girl* and *Agape* represent the balance we need to move forward: disruption and compassion. One charges through the gates. The other holds the line. Both are essential if we are going to change the world.

If we want a food system that reflects our values—not just our appetites—we have to make room for that balance. We need farmers growing food that heals. We need systems that support real transition. And we need to stop rewarding destruction while those who choose a better way are left behind.

There's a verse in Hosea 2:18 that says:

*"I will make a covenant for them with the beasts of the field, the birds in the sky, and the creatures that move along the ground… so that all may lie down in safety."*

That's not just scripture—it's a roadmap. It's the future we're here to build.

Rowdy Girl and Agape's stories remind me that the work we do must ripple far beyond the fences of Rowdy Girl Sanctuary. Because that ripple must become a wave. And that wave—when carried with reverence, clarity, and wisdom—*becomes the ocean.*

An ocean deeper than anything we've ever known.

And it is in the unknown that the truth lives.

We must be willing to go there—because that's where we've *never* been.

And it's where we've never been that *everything* can change.

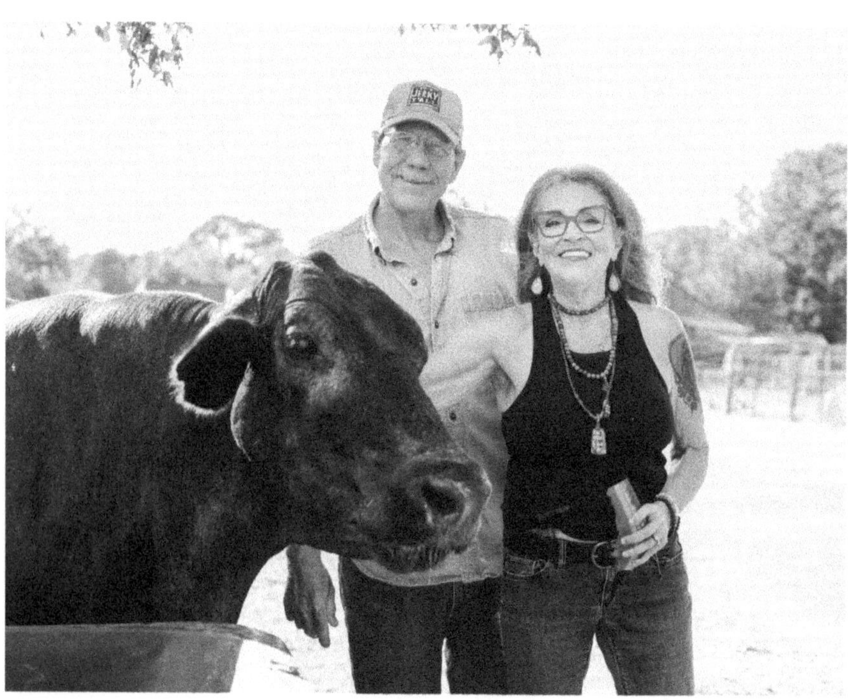

**Figure 13 Renée, Tommy, and Agape**. *Agape was a miracle—a mother scarred by loss who rose into the herd's matriarch. As her sight dimmed, her trust grew. She spent her last years in peace, leaving this world knowing she was loved.*

# *Conclusion: A Call to Action*

Once you see the truth, you can't unsee it. The same system that turns mothers into a "supply chain" is the one that sold me a lie—until I loved Rowdy Girl like my own child. That love ripped the veil away. I saw a new reality, and there was no going back.

*There's a door that we dare not go through, because if we do we will see that all of the animals are just like us.*

But once you walk through, you're forever changed. That's why some of us risk arrest to show the truth. Ag-Gag laws and labels like "humane" and "organic" are part of the cover-up. And that's why I'm not here to just end factory farming. I'm here to end all animal farming.

My AA sponsor calls me her "little Moses" because I will walk through obstacles most people call impossible. That's how I crossed my own Red Sea—and it's how we will cross this sea of lies together. Not with a staff, but with our voices. One voice will become a resounding chorus.

We are addicted—to violence, to the killing machine, and then we spoon-feed it to our children. To top it off, we are being factory farmed ourselves. But going vegan for the animals breaks the cycle. It wakes you up.

When you wake up, you can't stay silent.

**Say out loud**: *This must end.* **Refuse right now:** to put chopped-up bodies on your plate. **Witness** the suffering and speak against it—*quietly, loudly, and boldly every day, every minute, every breath you take!*

We are all called to be a Moses in our own hometowns. **Say it with me:** *Set them free. Let them go.*

I'll be right there with you—in thought, word, and deed—raising our rowdy voices until the cows come home.

# Appendix: The Eight Limbs of Yoga

1. Yamas (self-control and how we live in the world)
   - Ahimsa (nonviolence)
   - Satya (truth)
   - Asteya (non-stealing)
   - Brahmacharya (non-indulgence)
   - Aparigraha (non-possessiveness)
2. Niyamas (how we relate to ourselves)
   - Saucha (cleanliness)
   - Santosha (contentment)
   - Tapas (self-discipline)
   - Swadhyaya (self-study)
   - Ishvara pranidhana (connection with divinity)
3. Asana (yoga poses)
4. Pranayama (the practice of awareness using the breath)
5. Pratyahara (withdrawal from the senses)
6. Dharana (concentration)
7. Dhyana (meditation)
8. Samadhi (freedom from illusion)

Patañjali, *The Yoga Philosophy with Comments of Bhojaraja*, edited by Tookaram Tatya, translated by J. R. Ballantyne and Govind Shastri Deva (Bombay: Theosophical Publication Fund, 1882; final revised edition, 1885).

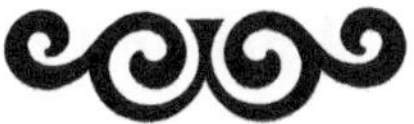

# *Notes*

## Chapter 1

1 Laura Bennet et al., "Waking Up Too Early—the Consequences of Preterm Birth on Sleep Development," *Journal of Physiology* 596, no. 23 (December 2018): 5687–708, accessed November 13, 2025, https://pmc.ncbi.nlm.nih.gov/articles/PMC6265542/. (pmc.ncbi.nlm.nih.gov).

## Chapter 7

1 Bill W., *Alcoholics Anonymous: The Story of How Many Thousands of Men and Women Have Recovered from Alcoholism* (New York: Alcoholics Anonymous World Services, 2001).

## Chapter 12

1 Sadhguru, "The Three Fundamental Nadis—Ida, Pingala and Sushumna," Isha Wisdom, May 6, 2013, accessed November 13, 2025, https://isha.sadhguru.org/en/wisdom/article/the-three-fundamental-nadis.

2 Arthur Avalon (Sir John Woodroffe), *The Serpent Power: The Secrets of Tantric and Shaktic Yoga* (London: Luzac & Co., 1919).

## Chapter 13

1 Will Tuttle, *The World Peace Diet* (New York: Lantern Books, 2005).

## Chapter 17

1 "Red Trailer," YouTube video, 2:15, posted by "RedTrailers9792," August 14, 2014, accessed November 13, 2025, https://www.youtube.com/watch?v=QP9EwvgoD48.

## Chapter 19

1 Alcoholics Anonymous, *Alcoholics Anonymous: The Story of How Many Thousands of Men and Women Have Recovered from Alcoholism*, 4th ed. (New York: Alcoholics Anonymous World Services, 2002).

2 Kip Andersen and Kameron Waters, *Christspiracy: The Spirituality Secret*, documentary film, 2024; trailer posted March 5, 2024, YouTube video, 2:21, accessed November 13, 2025, https://www.youtube.com/watch?v=PlHaV5rEBN8.

## Chapter 20

1 Wayne W. Dyer, *You'll See It When You Believe It* (New York: William Morrow, 1989).

## Chapter 21

1 "Rescue Ranch," YouTube video, accessed November 13, 2025, https://www.youtube.com/watch?v=RrvZXyosYwA.

## Chapter 24

1 Andrea J. Garmyn et al., "More Than Meat: Contributions of Livestock Systems Beyond Meat Production," *Animal Front* 11, no. 2 (May 2021): 4, citing Ritchie and Poser (FAO), accessed November 13, 2025, https://pmc.ncbi.nlm.nih.gov/articles/PMC8127679/.

2 Gabriel Cousens, "Home," Tree of Life Center US, accessed November 13, 2025, https://treeoflifecenterus.com/.

3 *Conscious Lifestyle Magazine*, accessed November 13, 2025, https://consciouslifestylemag.com/.

4 *One Green Planet*, accessed November 13, 2025, https://www.onegreenplanet.org/.

# Chapter 26

1 "Farm Drama in Newfane as Protesters Calling for the Return of Cows," *WKBW*, July 27, 2022, accessed November 13, 2025, https://www.wkbw.com/news/local-news/farm-drama-in-newfane-as-protesters-calling-for-the-return-of-cows?utm_source=chatgpt.com.

# Chapter 29

1 "TV Quality Turkey Rescue CHI CHI & ALANA," YouTube video, 5:24, posted by Chee Wei Productions, February 12, 2024, accessed November 13, 2025, https://youtu.be/wZkAJtIJCSU.

2 Rebecca Olds, "How Many Turkeys Are Killed for Thanksgiving?," *Deseret News*, November 18, 2023, accessed November 13, 2025, https://www.deseret.com/2023/11/18/23950898/how-many-turkeys-are-killed-each-year-for-thanksgiving/.

3 Dr. Sailesh Rao, "Dr. Sailesh Rao," *Climate Healers*, accessed November 13, 2025, https://climatehealers.org/sailesh-rao.

4 "How Healing Ourselves Heals the Planet," *Plant Based Curious* podcast episode, iHeartRadio, accessed November 13, 2025, https://www.iheart.com/podcast/269-plant-based-curious-110759600/episode/how-healing-ourselves-heals-the-planet-271318983/.

# Chapter 30

1 Omri Wallach, "How Big Is the U.S. Cheese Stockpile?," *Visual Capitalist*, October 23, 2022, accessed November 13, 2025, https://www.visualcapitalist.com/us-cheese-stockpile/.

2 Scot M. Miller et al., "Anthropogenic Emissions of Methane in the United States," *Proceedings of the National Academy of Sciences* 110, no. 50 (October 18, 2013).

3 "Livestock's Long Shadow: Environmental Issues and Options," 2006, Food and Agriculture Organization of the United Nations, https://www.fao.org/3/a0701e/a0701e.pdf.

4 "Ag Payments Tracker Stats," Agriculture Fairness Alliance, accessed November 13, 2025, https://www.agriculturefairnessalliance.org/ag-tracker-stats/ag-payments-tracker.

# Chapter 31

1 "Livestock Forage Disaster Program (LFP)," US Department of Agriculture, Farm Service Agency (FSA), https://www.fsa.usda.gov/resources/programs/livestock-forage-disaster-program-lfp; "Livestock Indemnity Program (LIP)," US Department of Agriculture, Farm Service Agency (FSA), https://www.fsa.usda.gov/programs-and-services/disaster-assistance-program/livestock-indemnity.

2 "Noninsured Disaster Assistance Program (NAP)," US Department of Agriculture, Farm Service Agency (FSA), https://www.fsa.usda.gov/resources/programs/noninsured-disaster-assistance-program-nap.

3 "Farm Subsidy Database," Environmental Working Group (EWG), https://farm.ewg.org/; Christopher Leonard, *The Meat Racket: The Secret Takeover of America's Food Business* (New York: Simon & Schuster, 2014).

# Chapter 32

1 Beyond Meat, "Planting Change: Challenging the Status Quo," YouTube video, 9:55, May 20, 2021 (approx.), accessed November 13, 2025, https://www.youtube.com/watch?v=fEThKT1MPKM.

2 Samara Mendez and William McAuliffe, "Effects of Restrictive Animal Product Alternative Labeling Laws on Supply-Chain Costs," *Rethink Priorities*, January 24, 2025, accessed November 13, 2025, https://rethinkpriorities.org/research-area/effects-of-restrictive-animal-product-alternative-labeling-laws-on-supply-chain-costs/.

# *Resources*

## Words That Inspired My Vegan Journey


1 *The Way to the Kingdom*, by Joseph Sieber Benner (originally published 1932).

2 *The Brother of Jesus and the Lost Teachings of Christianity*, by Jeffrey J. Bütz (Rochester, VT: Inner Traditions, 2005).

3 *Your Hope of Glory: The Life and Teachings of Jesus*, Elizabeth Sand Turner (Kansas City, MO: Unity School of Christianity, 1959).

4 *Jesus and the Essenes*, by Dolores Cannon (Huntsville, AR: Ozark Mountain Publishing, 1999).

5 *The Essene Gospel of Peace*, Books 1–4, trans. by Edmond Bordeaux Szekely (Santa Barbara, CA: DeVorss & Co., 1926).

6 *Why Every Christian Should Be Vegan*, by Steve Heinze (Richmond, CA: House of Peace Publishing, 2012).

7 *A History of God*, by Karen Armstrong (New York: Ballantine Books, 1993).

8 *Forbidden Mysteries of Enoch*, by J. J. van der Leeuw (New York: Samuel Weiser, 1972).

9 *The Lost Teachings of Jesus*, Vol. 1, by Timothy Freke (New York: Sterling, 2001).

10 *The Lost Years of Jesus*, by Elizabeth Clare Prophet (New York: Summit University Press, 1994).

11 *Jesus' Audience*, by J. Duncan M. Derrett (New York, NY: Seabury Press, 1972).

12 *All That You Are*, by Paramahansa Yogananda (Los Angeles, CA: Self-Realization Fellowship, 1995).

13 *Lessons in Truth*, by H. Emilie Cady (Los Angeles, CA: Unity School of Christianity, 1896).

14 *A Course in Miracles*, Foundation for Inner Peace (San Francisco, CA: Foundation for Inner Peace, 1975).

15 *Alcoholics Anonymous: The Story of How Many Thousands of Men and Women Have Recovered from Alcoholism*, 4th ed. (New York: Alcoholics Anonymous World Services, 2002).

16 *The Book of Mormon* (Salt Lake City, UT: The Church of Jesus Christ of Latter-day Saints, 1981).

17 *The Living Gita*, by Swami Prabhupada (Los Angeles, CA: Bhaktivedanta Book Trust, 1986).

18 *The Yoga Sutras of Patanjali*, trans. by Swami Satchidananda (Buckingham, VA: Integral Yoga Publications, 1978).

19 *Sacred Nitnem* (Amritsar, India: SGPC, 2002).

20 *The Guru Granth Sahib*, ed. and trans. by Dr. Gopal Singh (Amritsar, India: SGPC, 2000).

21 *Tao Te Ching*, trans. by Stephen Mitchell (New York: HarperCollins, 1988).

22 *I Ching*, trans. by Richard Wilhelm and C. F. Baynes, ed. Cary F. Baynes (Princeton, NJ: Princeton University Press, 1967).

23 *The Apocrypha* (New York: Oxford University Press, 1991).

24 *The Vegan Bible*, by Virginia Messina (New York: Da Capo Press, 2019).

# Index

# *About the Author*

**Renée King-Sonnen** once believed her calling was to be a country-and-western singer and performer. She did not yet know that her voice was being prepared for a deeper reckoning—one that would begin on a Texas cattle ranch, where a single cow revealed the truth she had never questioned and shattered the world she thought she understood.

Renée is the founder of Rowdy Girl Sanctuary, the first documented beef cattle ranch in the world to go vegan and become a sanctuary for rescued farmed animals. What began as a personal moral awakening became a public testimony shaped by daily proximity to the animals whose lives reoriented her own.

Her story was captured in the documentary *Rowdy Girl*, which has screened internationally and reached audiences through PBS and other streaming platforms. Her story has reached millions worldwide, inviting a radical reexamination of animals, food, faith, and conscience.

Today, Renée speaks carrying the collective witness of cows and other farmed animals—amplifying lives long rendered invisible and inviting a profound reexamination of humanity's moral inheritance. She lives in Texas with her husband, Tommy, and the animals who continue to guide her work.